Recent Updates in Eating Disorders

Edited by Ignacio Jáuregui-Lobera and José Vicente Martínez-Quiñones

Published in London, United Kingdom

Recent Updates in Eating Disorders
http://dx.doi.org/10.5772/intechopen.100839
Edited by Ignacio Jáuregui-Lobera and José Vicente Martínez-Quiñones

Contributors
Farzaneh Saeedzadeh Sardahaee, Nasreddine Aissaoui, Lamia Hamaizia, Said Khalfa Mokhtar Brika, Ahmed Laamari, Ignacio Jáuregui-Lobera, José Vicente Martínez-Quiñones, José María Otín-del Castillo, Val Bellman, Amra Ćatović, Juan José Labora González, Pablo Soto-Casás

First published in London, United Kingdom, 2023 by IntechOpen
IntechOpen is the global imprint of INTECHOPEN LIMITED, registered in England and Wales, registration number: 11086078, 5 Princes Gate Court, London, SW7 2QJ, United Kingdom

British Library Cataloguing-in-Publication Data
A catalogue record for this book is available from the British Library

Additional hard and PDF copies can be obtained from orders@intechopen.com

Recent Updates in Eating Disorders
Edited by Ignacio Jáuregui-Lobera and José Vicente Martínez-Quiñones
p. cm.
Print ISBN 978-1-80356-521-7
Online ISBN 978-1-80356-522-4
eBook (PDF) ISBN 978-1-80356-523-1

Meet the editors

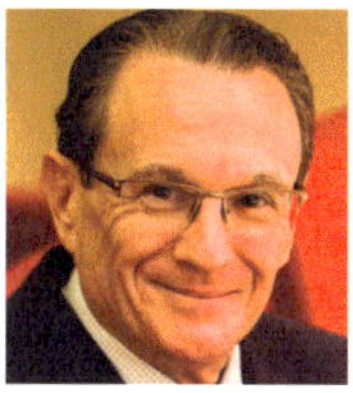

Ignacio Jáuregui-Lobera, MD, PsyD, MSc, directs the postgraduate course in Eating Disorders and Obesity at Pablo de Olavide University (Seville, Spain) and has been director of the Behavioural Science Institute and associate professor at the same university. He has worked as a psychiatrist, family practitioner, and psychologist in the field of eating disorders and obesity since 1993. He is the author of several books and book chapters and more than 100 scientific articles. He is an Academician of the Royal Academies of Medicine in Seville and Valladolid (Spain) and a member of the editorial boards of several international journals.

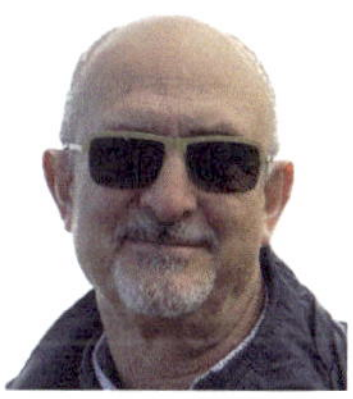

José Vicente Martínez Quiñones, MD, Ph.D., received his specialist training in neurosurgery at the Gómez Ulla Central Defense Hospital, Madrid. Since 2002 he has been developing his professional, teaching, and research activity at the MAZ Hospital in Zaragoza. He is an active member of the Spanish Societies of Neurosurgery, Neurology and Neurospine, and the Study Group for Spinal Diseases (GEER). He is the co-author of numerous popular medical books, co-author of book chapters, and author/co-author of original medical articles in national and international journals. He has participated in more than 100 presentations at various national and international conferences and has been involved in research projects both at the community level and in the national R&D Plan.

Contents

Preface

Recent Updates in Eating Disorders aims to raise recent relevant issues about eating disorders and obesity. We talk about an 'eating disorder society' insofar as it constitutes a constellation of eating behaviours and practices conducive to the development of these pathologies. During adolescence, the most vulnerable stage of life, this constellation facilitates the presence of risk situations which often neither the individuals nor their families are able to detect. It is important to be aware of behaviours that occur before the emergence of an eating disorder. While there are factors that facilitate the development of anorexia or bulimia nervosa, the other side of the coin is the problem of obesity, from childhood onwards, in all types of societies, whether more or less prosperous.

From a clinical perspective, it is important to bear in mind the epidemiological aspects of these disorders, and to consider their presence in males, which is not always well reflected in the literature. It is important to talk not only about diagnostic criteria but also about severity criteria and the presence of comorbidity, in order to establish better protocols for therapeutic action. Aspects such as exercise or the question of sexual orientation must be taken into account.

Another very relevant issue today is that different eating patterns can have a negative or positive influence on the development of eating disorders as well as overweight and obesity. Alterations in eating patterns clearly point to one disorder or the other. Sudden changes in eating habits, especially in adolescents, are often an indicator of the onset of an eating disorder.

Finally, we want to address the issue of social media networks and their influence on the development of eating disorders (and many other problems). As one of the authors rightly points out, social media are now a major socialisation factor in the lives of adolescents, who make intensive use of them to relate to each other and to the world. This has led to a great deal of scientific research on the influence of this medium of communication in many areas of the life and development of adolescents, especially on their physical and mental health. We review relevant psychological phenomena associated with the use of social networks in order to understand their influence on adolescent behaviour, recent research on the main psychosocial risk factors for problematic internet use by this age group and their possible relationship with eating disorders, and proposals adopted within the European Union and in Spain for the control of harmful content on the internet, especially that by apologists for anorexia and bulimia, which until very recently escaped any possibility of control despite their importance for public health. The potential of technology to implement adequate controls is discussed, and a research project is presented for the detection and neutralisation of eating disorder apologist postings on Twitter, financed and implemented by the APE Foundation with the collaboration of the University of Zaragoza, Spain.

While this work is neither exhaustive nor extensive, we nevertheless hope it will be of interest and will open up further lines of study and research in the near future.

Ignacio Jáuregui-Lobera
Pablo de Olavide University,
Sevilla, Spain

José Vicente Martínez-Quiñones
Hospital MAZ,
Zaragoza, Spain

Section 1

Epidemiology

Chapter 1

The Eating Disorder's Society

Juan José Labora González and Pablo Soto-Casás

Abstract

Feeding has been subjected to a process of medicalization throughout history that has caused its perception to be assimilated to the intake of nutrients. However, it is necessary to conceive feeding as a total social phenomenon. That is to say, a phenomenon that impregnates food and the practices that surround it with different meanings. It is therefore necessary to understand how certain social dynamics (secularization, rationalization, bureaucratization) have modified the way we feed ourselves and how we interpret food itself. This, in turn, has generated a series of negative meanings that have influenced how we perceive the body and the image of people. The calculability of nutrients and an unrealistic and unattainable image canon for people have been installed. Thus, a social food imaginary has been created based on a whole series of myths that are transmitted through social networks and that produce that the society in which we live has become an obesogenic and lipophobic society. It is therefore necessary to understand how the social imaginary of fat and fatness has been constructed in order to understand how people perceive their body image and how this can be altered.

Keywords: eating disorders, social imaginaries, body, feeding, society

1. Introduction

> *The human sciences, since a long time ago, they are insisting on the fact that the human feeding belongs to an imaginary, symbolic and social dimension (...). It is a commonplace: we are feeding ourselves from nourishment, but also from the imagination [1].*

In this chapter, we are going to understand the pacing throughout the feeding process. This process must be analyzed like a social phenomenon, which acquires identity dimensions with people, and it is affecting in a great scale by moral aspects which affect mainly how obesity and fat is understood. Therefore, in the feeding process, we should acknowledge phenomenon like the fasting, hunger, diet, food taboo, etc.

Furthermore, we will explain how the important process of medicalization of the feeding resulted into a reduction of the feeding phenomenon by the fact of acquiring necessary nourishments for surviving (diet/nutrition). This locates the symbolic power for its social evaluation again in the hands of doctors.

In fact, the food and its social uses were soon associated with different social meanings. The symbolic universe of the feeding was branding this practice from the beginning of the times. The Anthropology linked the practice of the feeding with taboo, the totemist, and the sacrifice [2]. The taboo, at the same time, it was linked to the impurity's meaning of the soil where everyone should stand apart from it [3]. Some foods, as like Harris would say [4], they are healthy for eating, and there are others that are not. In such rules, the Sociology interprets them as part of the symbolic universe of each society and/or culture. From this perspective, the forbidden consumption of beef in India, or some specific cultures that were allowing cannibalism in different ages since the prehistorical times, like it was founded in Atapuerca, the Tupinambo in Brazil in the sixteenth century, the Yanomami on the border between this and Venezuela until practically today, the Aztecs in the sixteenth century, the Fore in the highlands of New Guinea until the end of the twentieth century, etc. [5, 6].

It was Marcel Mauss [7] who was the first to recognize feeding as the category of total social fact. This category implied, to the French sociologist that feed would be turned into a speaker of institutions: religious, legal, economic and moral (we understand that this sphere would include the politics and the family). All in all, we eat what we are. Thinking from the same framework, Herrera would say that "far from being a spectre, from the beginning, a simple sign of other fact, the feeding is the social act where memory and fashion are intertwined, arguing and practice, power and knowledge, liking and necessity; where all the references are added, where behaviours are defined, where the differences are established" [8].

This starting point imposes the necessity of performing an analysis of the social dynamics that affects feeding. In specific, the medicalization process is the same, the canon of beauty that rule with an iron hand the postmodern societies and the obesity phenomena. This is understood from the perspective that the feeding as a phenomenon that is born and produces, in specific types of moral that can allow to introduce unique meanings in social imaginaries that we share, not only with the workers that we work with people with eating disorders (onwards, ED), but also with them.

2. The medicalization of the feeding

Following Fischler, the relationship between the medicine and the feeding is inseparable, hence, "feeding is the first step to access to the body, namely, a privileged instrument of medical intervention. The incarnation explains the difference between the dietetic and cooks some kind of continuum, ambiguity, may be a fundamental rivalry" [1]. From Hippocratic medicine the medical treatment seems linked to some specific ways of eating. The Hippocratic medicine was based on the necessity of achieving the mood balance and in order to, in a sickness situation -we mean, an unbalanced situation-, the food was employed as a medium or tools for the doctor's work.

Nevertheless, in the prehistory of the society of the hunter-gathering they dedicated a huge amount of daily energy for seeking food. They hunted what they could with weapons that they had. Women, however, they recollected plants and edible seeds as a way of complement the diet. They were having satiety or relativity abundance and other of famine and even starvation. This situation was the main characteristic of the nomad lifestyle that they had. After a while, agriculture emerged that, namely, allowed to evolve into a new sedentary life. However, this fact did not prevent famine, whether it was for climate reasons or for other kind (plagues, lack of insecticides, etc.) The last mayor famines in the occidental world can be situated in France between 1741 and 1742 and Ireland between 1846 and 1848 due to the lack of potatoes [1].

In the present times, starvation continues to exist in the world, but it usually affects the majority of the population of the Third World, or the so-called undeveloped countries, as it is said in the politically correct paradigm likes to call them. Countries for known structural global causes, they do not achieve that wished development that emerged in international analysis or in macro figures that, unfortunately, are not edible and they do not redistribute, most of the times, a redistribution of the wealth which is still located in a small number of people.

Anyway, Herrera [8] points out that from the XVII in advanced it will raise the process of the blossoming of the modern nourishment. This process of modifying the feeding for the contemporary society would be characterized by the following traits: it is a process of a progressive secularization, rationality and bureaucracy. However, what it is true if that the act of feeding, always was affected by a number of tensions:

- The tension between the good and evil. Since the surge of different cultures, some foods were affected by morality (disgust, taboo, etc.); determinate by different cultures or religions. For instance, the prohibition of eating pork for Muslims, or eating beef for Indian o the disgust for occidentals for eating snakes or insects.

- The tension for eating for pleasure or for ethical reasons, morality or religion.

- The tension between moderation and gluttony.

Some authors [8, 9] point out that this tension "were resolved" by gathering around the process of a progressive calculated rationalization and leaded by nutrition, for ending being assumed by the homonymous medical knowledge. If in the antiquity the argument for recommending one or other food choice were clearly biased due to moral factors linked to religion or social, moral, with the irruption of nutrition the social speeches allow to estimate what kind of food is correct for each person in specific. Or what food would be beneficial for a specific person to eat, hence it may be harmful in that case.

Using the Foucauldian terminology, Coveney [9] would say that the apparition of the nutrition was due to the fact of the rationality feeding that was produced by the workhouses and prisons. These possibilities broad up a new kind of governmentality allowed by the surge of Social Science's applied statistics and the Medicine.

Despite of this exquisite asepsis in discourses, some authors warn us that maybe behind of the façade we could find that these discourses are "equally "pastorals" in their intentions and objectives" [9]. In this sense, the author claims that "the nutrition is not only a science, but also an ethos" [9]. Diet, then, would be defined by the formula [9]:

$$\text{Diet} = \text{Health} + \text{Medicine} + \text{Lifestyle}. \quad (1)$$

Some specific social dynamics: the rising of the population, the rapid acceleration of lifestyle, the women's incorporation to the workforce, etc., it forced the necessity of acquiring food in the most rapid way (with the minimum time expended) and the minimum effort (minimum economic and energy cost); it is imposed that what it is called Fordist diet [10]. At the same time, this process leads to a *macdonalization* [11], namely, a system that responds to the population demands. A system that favors the efficiency, allowing a fasting feeding (both in relation to the raw material, as the elaboration process, as the price that is charged to the population that consume them).

Some processes or social changes can be pointed out in order to influence, the changes of the feeding habits in the contemporaneity [8]:

- The progressive urbanization and industrialization that was produced in twentieth century.
- The globalization.
- The women joining the workforce.
- The regulation and time distribution dedicated to work and the consequences of incrementing the time destined to leisure time.
- The mass population schooling. The demographics are changing, led by the birth-rate reduction and the population aging.
- The changes are produced in the ideas and values: the imaginaries of the body, the new beauty standards, the resignification of the obese, the ecological movement, the new feeding consumption habits: vegan, vegetarian, ecological products, light products, etc.
- The individualization that characterizes contemporary societies in the field of food causes people to see themselves "drowned" by the need to make responsible decisions taken in the mare magnum of contradictory information about the characteristics of food. In addition to this, the media that offers information and the advertisements is increasing even more the typical characteristics of scientific jargon, what it turns to be the common framework for talking about; Omega 3, triglycerides, cholesterol HDL or LDL, active bifidus, etc. and a huge panoply of modified food with the supposed benefits of characteristics which are found to be really difficult for the casual consumer understanding them; milk with more calcium than normal, light products, drinks for lowing the cholesterol levels, foods for improving the student's memory, etc.

All these possibilities are immense which they produce "an informative cacophony where the ignorance of products and the processes of the elaborating food (...) the modern commensal it is plunged into a permanent state of insecurity and uncertainty where there are no reliable criteria or coherent rationality funding their decisions" [8].

These changes in society cause food to undergo a series of changes [8, 12, 13]:

- In the cultural representations and the symbolic value of the food: the fat consideration, the feeding taboos, etc.
- In the rules, consuming options: homogenization of consuming (types of food, ways of preparing, etc.), the *macdonalization*, the unfocused of the feeding, the timelessness, disocialization, the offshoring of the meals.

- In the ways of learning and transmission of knowledge and feeding skills: contest and reality shows, etc.
- In the feeding language: the spherification, textures, the trompe l'oeil, deconstruction of dishes, etc.
- In the values and worries related to the feeding: the health care (level of glucose and cholesterol), the overweight worry, the quest for thinness, etc.
- The knowledge and feeding abilities of the population.
- The foods democratization originated by the rising gastronomy situation [1].

This type of changes and dynamics created a paradoxical eating defined from two incompatible characteristics: the homogeneity of the feeding and the diet [1, 2] and the food diversity and cuisines that currently coexist [8].

2.1 The feeding and the risk of the ED

Nonetheless, what is the link between the feeding with the ED? In this case, this hinge concept is the consideration from the Sociology in the contemporary societies, such as the risk society [14–17].

As far as food is concerned, the legal regulations that the food industry must respect are increasingly strict. This raises the risk perception among the population, something that was ate until it may be harmful and must be retired from the market. Secondly, new debates are emerging:

> *Regarding bioethics about the genetic alteration of the foods, the environmental degradation which involves the organization of production and the technological apps or the nutritional degradation of the own food (lack of fiber, vitamins, high fat content, sugar and salt, excess questionable chemical compounds...) they are creating perceptions and risk situations to the consumers that demand the introduction of strict regulations that guarantees the food security [8].*

These kinds of characterizations produce that the health field is not only restricted to effective health and real, otherwise it enhances their limits until reaching the potential health. Now, in addition to the diseases that they suffer, it matters as well as the risk factors, the predispositions related to the risk situation, etc. The sanitary prevention just started to enter into our lives.

In the present times being sick is not the same, you have to be vigilant in order to maintain your health in a good shape. From time to time you will have to measure your vascular pressure, be aware of the glucose levels, if she is a woman, she would have to get a mammogram, if he is a man he would have to get a prostate check... This is how we enter in a long list of "mandatory" individual actions that we have to assume as responsible people. The sanitary prevention can turn into one of the monsters that threatens our individual freedom along with the internet (and the possible elimination of our privacy) or even the flexisecurity paradigm (which justify any domain measure of our bodies and our mobility freedom despite of being consecrated in almost any of existing Magna carta).

This calculability that characterized the social imaginary of nutrition opens the door to the social evaluations in another sense. Right now, each person can know what the recommended food intake is, for healthy in their specific case. That is, for me it can be 1500 calories, for another person 2000 calories, etc. If I eat more than is recommended, evaluations automatically appear that say that I do not have enough willpower, or I am an indolent person, or that I am simply fat because I decide to be (guilt), etc. Fatness becomes governed and leaded by a calculative logic [18], which frames everything in the sphere of morality.

In addition, the definition of the frameworks that sets the limits to the mentioned assessments is established by the medical staff. And they are transmitted to society due to the guarantee of medical research. Herrera reminds us that "Doctors, biologists, educators, publicists, media, national and international institutions...are now claimed as information agents and educators in the food field, becoming an integral part -and often decisive- of an agri-food system that is thus significantly enlarged in its elements" [8]. And what this sociologist calls rational superstition, that is, "a new sacredness that institutes faith in scientific rationality, and its legitimate administration by a medical priesthood" [8].

Once again Herrera will be the one who sums up in a magnificent way the situation of food in contemporary societies when they say that:

> *The main consequence of the process of rationalization in culinary practices is observed in the radical change of agency that entails. The progressive extension of medical-biological rationality, and the consequent erosion of traditional religious restrictions and patterns of social distinction, of the dictates of the body and of tradition, induces a growing reversal of the agenda in the subjects of food that figures in the transition from eating to nutrition, from action to reception, from the attribution of an agent role for the diner related to a patient role [8].*

Based on the introduction of morality in the food imaginary, the question is whether this provoked some kind of consequence or influence in the field of ED. As a matter of fact, it does. Gracia-Arnáiz and Comelles [19] refer that the biological. Medical paradigm imposes a threefold look at medical practice: The medical-centrism, that is, the use of a reductionist rationality supposedly shielded by the scientific asepsis, androcentrism and misogyny.

The process of medicalization of food takes its first steps in the famous "experiment" carried out at the spa of Battle Creek in Michigan in 1863 and that would end in an experience of creating a healthy diet for the human being, but that along the way was commodified and led to the famous cereals Kellogg's [9, 20]. This process takes off after the Second World War, guided by the attempt to reduce the levels of cholesterol, glucose, etc., but it will do so by establishing the parameter of statistical normality established by medicine. Toro notes that in the United States "By 1880 girls were conspicuously worried about not looking too thin" [20]. And Gracia-Arnáiz and Comelles qualify that "Preventing obesity was never a biomedical priority before the twentieth century. Being fat was not considered pathological, malnutrition, yes" [19].

These types of events run parallel to the change in the canon of beauty. Referents such as Marilyn Monroe or Sofía Loren are abandoned and the canon evolves towards the image of the Twiggy model [19, 20]. From that moment on, the aforementioned model will be followed by: Kate Moss, Nieves Álvarez, Cindy Crawford, etc. But perhaps it would not hurt to remember that all these women, over time, ended up recognizing their eating disorders or, at least, dalliances with inappropriate eating behaviors.

Right now, the problem of the image is much more complex, because programs like Photoshop allow to create women and men that do not exist and will never exist. People with perfect images that only exist in the virtual reality of the computer documents in which they are stored and edited.

All this outlines a social imaginary permeated by a true mythology that, following Sanders and Bazalgette [21] would respond to the following myths:

- All kinds of fat in food are bad.
- The roundness is not healthy.
- Thinness is healthy.
- Fatness or fat can be lost quickly, and this is not dangerous.
- There is a special type of fat that occurs in women, called cellulite.
- Cellulite fat is caused by toxins.
- You can reduce the fat of a particular part of the body, for example, hips and thighs.
- Certain foods and certain combinations can activate metabolism and accelerate weight loss. In this sense, the Dukan diet is fashionable lately, based on the predominant protein intake.
- Women under 50 are at risk for heart disease.
- Dieting is healthy.

Toro after making a tour of the investigations that studied the dissatisfaction of people with his body, concludes that "practically all citizens value his physical appearance, pays attention to it, thinks about it, worries and tries to modify it actively" [20]. In relation to this matter, Moreno finds three types of beliefs that would lay the basis of what he calls "ideologies about eating disorders" [22].

- The belief in the existence of a single body market that would not be affected: the social class, the phase of the life cycle, or the life choices that people take.
- Even if a specific model exists, each individual would make a personal retranslation based on his or her body "diagnosis".
- By becoming the body in modernity on the battlefield of its own construction one can believe that this presents no limit. Opposing to this, Moreno points out that the aforementioned battlefield can transfer the confrontation to the perception that would swing between maximizing the problem of the body and the "Belief that the same is an exaggeration cultivated by professionals eager to read in the key of pathology in everyday life" [8]

In his research he concludes that the social position of the individual determines in a similar way his perception that in the case of EA "the body as a possible space of a personal construction project is absent from the discourse" [22]. Moreno [22] detects the resistance of the influence of discourses in the symbolic sphere of the body in certain sectors of the population:

- In men, especially if they are married. It is also the case that "among men, as we decrease socially, the number of cases that people consider normal increases" [22].
- In the elderly (70 years).
- In people whose perception tilts towards the material consideration of the body (the solidity of the body would make it difficult to modify it).
- In the people of the urban habitat.

Compared to the above enumeration, the social sectors most likely trend to influence their body perception, like middle-aged women, around 45 years old would be [22], in specific, women who reside in small localities (less than 5000 inhabitants). Overall, according to Moreno [22] women would show a greater tendency to show perceptions of having a higher-than-normal weight.

3. The moralization: obesogenic and lipophobic societies

One of the most repeated expressions in the scientific literature to describe the ED would be to define them as an epidemic of contemporary societies [23, 24]. This occurs in parallel to the consideration of current societies as societies suffering from the obesity epidemic [25]. As a result, different authors have been using the term lipophobia [1, 26, 27] to describe the current situation of hate to fat, the fear of fattening produced by the process of medicalization of the body and food.

Lipophobia would be a relatively recent phenomenon, Gracia-Arnáiz tells us that:

> *Fatness was, and still is, welcomed in numerous societies. Gluttony and binge eating can be a socially accepted and even valued practice that not everyone can afford. In contexts where food shortages are not unusual, corpulent individuals were more likely to survive. While being thin was associated with fearsome diseases, being fat denoted status and often beauty and sexual appeal [26].*

What processes led us here? The truth is that some specialist [25] studying obesity, pointed out that its imaginaries were always paradoxical. In the Middle Ages, Vigarello distinguishes "between two possible looks. On the one hand, there is the fat that imposes its mass and causes an immediate respect, which provides distinction and holiness. And, on the other hand, the fatness that underlies its heaviness, which produces the grind and the weakness [25]. Thus, there would be a social imaginary of fatness, provided it does not impede the mobility of the person, characteristic of the upper classes. The nobility and the aristocracy were the social strata that enjoyed sufficient economic level to be able to afford to maintain a certain leisure and a high level of food intake, which together could produce excessive weight gain.

But from the end of the twelfth century and the beginning of the thirteenth two relevant phenomena occur. From that moment on the pastoral work of the monks who used to live more closed in their abbeys will increase. On the other hand, the growth of cities modified sociability, and facilitated the sermon itself, which would be supported by phenomena such as that of mendicant monks [25]. You have to control the appetite for food, as well as sexual appetite, abstinence and moderation, can protect us from falling into sin. As Coveney [9] points out, Christian practices are rearranged around eating habits, examination of conscience, confession and penance.

The food itself in this sense is an ambivalent element: it is a gift of God and as such should be considered; in addition to being used as an instrument of mortification of the body and praise of the divinity through fasting; but at the same time, carries with it great opportunities to fall into sin: food as something external that could contaminate the body. Fat participated in the canon of beauty of the moment. Vigarello [25] cites some excerpts from the romances of the time in which we speak of "tender and beautiful fatties" [25] and how in the "Roman de la Rose" a "feminine and beautiful maiden (who is) quite fat" is quoted [25]. But as Vigarello [25] says, fat was present until the fifteenth century in the discourse, but it was practically absent from the iconographic representation. Even some historical personage of which there is much news of his corpulence as William the Conqueror was represented without this characteristic. The fat in the image used to be reduced to the representation of a rounded belly, but it was not usually represented in the rest of the body. Obesity was structured around the popular/distinguished distinction [25]. It was therefore a social differentiation to which moral meanings are beginning to be assigned, but which will increasingly be pointed towards the moral sphere in later times.

At the same time, we find a medical discourse still vague and without concretion, and of a low level of influence [25]. In the Renaissance we find a revaluation of the possibility of activity. In the sixteenth century the criticism of the heavy, of the enormous, of laziness was introduced. But without forgetting that thinness is also criticized, the object of search is balance [25]. This equilibrium, which is attempting to recover from the classical canon that had been established in Greece centuries ago, is embodied in the man of Vitruvius, which Leonardo elevates to classical canon through the balance of the Aurea proportion. Leonardo recovers the classical canon of the Greek proportion that had defined the ratio between the body and the head in 7 to 1. But as exemplified by Raich, Sánchez Carracedo and López Guimerà [27], although the Venus de Milo meets the requirements of the aforementioned canon of beauty and balance, it would not meet those of the current canon, since the aforementioned statue would need a size 42. And such considerations will remain throughout history. Marilyn Monroe and Sofía Loren are cited in the literature as examples of the sixties beauty canon [20, 27]. It should be remembered that Marilyn responded to the canon of the famous 90–60-90, but in reality, Marilyn wore a size 44 [27]. So, the famous triple figure still dominates the popular imaginary, the truth is that it does not respond closely to the measurements of supermodels and advertising models today. The 90–60-90 parameter, applied today, would relegate figures such as the two actresses cited to be "seen as plump, low-muscled women" [27].

Even so, fatness was preferred to thinness. Thinness with its fat removal prevented reaching the balance that was the criterion of beauty. In addition, the thinness was linked to the classic type of melancholy described by the mood model [25]. At this time there are many engravings that reflect different allegories of melancholy. This emotion had already been pointed out by Aristotle in the famous problem n° 1 in Section XXX of his Problems [28] as a possible cause of mental illness. The etymology of melancholy itself refers to mélas (black) and khôle (bile) [29]. The predominance of black bile makes people unstable, but at the same time, it makes them capable of great works of intellectual or artistic character. This kind of link between melancholy and genius was picked up by Cicero and passed through him to the entire Western culture (Seneca Plutarco Galeno Marsilio Ficino Montaigne). Until being sanctioned by Diderot through its inclusion in the Encyclopedia when, on the other hand, it was something already installed in the popular culture of the time [30]. This link reaches to the present time in which some specialist relates the high IQ with a personality structure that generates emotional difficulties that affect the patterns of functioning of people in their daily lives [31].

This process will end in melancholy swallowed up by medicine because:

> *Within the process of medicalization and medicamentation of daily life, people learned to denominate as "depression" most of the problems of life (frustrations, disappointments, burdens, lack of happiness), so that the thresholds of acceptance of the "discomfort" and the ability to face life's vicissitudes normally was lost [32].*

The iconography finally begins to reflect large, greasy bodies, eager for reality and implantation in space [25]. One only must remember some of the figures painted by El Bosco. And not to mention the bodies painted by Rubens; to finish remembering the epitome of "las tres Gracias".

As usually happens in history, this moment of excess and lack of measure follows the time of the containment of bodies. This containment would occur at two levels: at the physical level with the systematization from the sixteenth and seventeenth centuries of the physical systems of containment of the female body: the corsets, the bodices, the slips, etc.; and at social level the first diets sprout from the imaginary dry mood. The fat is linked to the liquid. The diet should be carried out with the intake of meat, astringent foods, avoiding, on the contrary, typical birds of rainy climates or with stagnant waters, as well as legumes or citrus containing a lot of liquid [25]. The contemporary construction of obesity would take its first steps in the Enlightenment. It is at this time that the consideration of fatness is individualized. There will be as many fatties as individuals. Obesity becomes an object of the gaze: "This work of the gaze transformed perception: alerts were created, and fatness was noted that did not exist, concerns were displaced, the gaze was sharpened" [25].

We are at the moment when science is establishing the measures of length, weight, etc. This helped the establishment of two symbolic universes, which unfortunately still live with us today. These two universes would be concretized in particular in "two thresholds of "acceptance" of fatness. Towards 1780, the Galerie des modes points to a considerable reduction in the female size and a greater freedom of the male volume: the lightness of women opposes the density of men" [25]. The male model begins to be established on the basis of more permissive criteria, they are allowed a certain body volume, even being plump; they, on the contrary, must show stylized sizes, even exaggerated by the use of corsets.

At that time obesity was borne. The first use in French is found in the second edition of 1701 of Antoine Furetière's Dicionario, when the term was not mentioned in the first edition of 1690 [25]. The word is commented on in the medical entries of the Dictionary. The change necessary to begin the medicalization process occurs because "fat is no longer a simple quantitative excess that should prevent sobriety, but it is a disorder, an internal degradation that has progressions of his determinations" [25]. Soon after we found in the Encyclopedia obesity as a medical term.

With the passage of time a rationalizing logic and new calculative type is introduced [25]. The nineteenth century must weigh obesity, measure it, etc., we must reduce everything to figures. This will cause the bourgeois world to give itself the swollen belly and take a step further with the sanction of the romantic prototype.

In Romanticism lapels reach impossible sizes, men had to wear belts that gird their waist, the use of vests is imposed, etc. The criterion to reach is youth full of strength and embodied in a spiky body. In the case of women, the paradigm is established fragility, often linked to a sickly appearance. The pallor of the skin, promoted by the use of different cosmetics; and care not to be exposed to the sun. The dominant values are the delicacy, passivity [25]. The subject's imaginary in Romanticism could be summed up saying that:

> *Everything is sorrow, a kind of metaphysical loneliness, abysmal, in front of a strange world, more than strange, to suggest that one is out of place in his own family world, a foreigner without a homeland (...). What remains as a remedy (...) is to enjoy sorrow, that is, to turn sadness into a way of life and to recreate itself in melancholy, because, as is known, melancholy is the joy of sadness [32].*

As Lama [33] points out in the nineteenth century, the disease was introduced into the social imaginary of women. But not only did women join the disease, but this link was sometimes made with mental illness [34–36]. In literature and opera of the nineteenth century, the so-called Scenes of Madness are widespread. Scenes in which a woman tormented by circumstances and/or an impossible love fell into the nets of madness. So it happens in Hamlet de Ambroise Thomas (Á vos jeux...Partagez-vous mes fleurs...Et maintenant, ècoutez ma chanson), in Il Pirata de Bellini (¡Oh! S'io potessi...Col sorriso d'innocenza), in Anna Bolena de Donizetti (Piangete voi...al dolce guide lame casstel natío) or in Luccia di Lammermoor by the same composer (Il doce suono...Ardon gl'icensi).

Once the standardization process of the models and measures was finished, there were parameters for medical science set the goal for each. The first therapies to treat patients suffering from obesity arise: the burning of calories, spas, etc.

Everything is ready to begin the desperate and absurd race of contemporary society towards martyrdom. Vigarello writes that towards the beginning of the twentieth century there is a displacement of two stigmas:

> *The fat one is first of all someone who "eludes", who rejects thinness, who despises striving to take care of himself. His defect is abandonment, and his responsibility, an intimate fault (...). Failure takes on a new form, which reinforces not only the generalization of treatments, but also the rise of psychology (...). The obese is no longer just a fat man. He is also incapable of changing: a failed identity [25].*

The medical imaginary of fat, therefore, aims to highlight the individual responsibility in the causality of this situation, forgetting the variety of influences and interactions: metabolic, genetic, and hormonal that can affect the obesity of people. All this causes a perception of obesity to be generated within medical science, which following Gracia-Arnáiz [26], is dominated by moral interpretations.

Obesity rapidly progressed from a social situation, a personal characteristic, to being considered a medical problem. This medical condition would, in turn, go from being considered a risk factor, to a disease, even an epidemic of global proportions [26]. When talking about obesity, unfortunately, we must begin by noting that this is not an ED, it is not classified as such either in the DSM or in the CIE. As a result of this it cannot be said to be a mental disorder. The surprising thing is to find in the literature articles that question this type of assertions, and that link obesity with a deranged gesture of eating that, ultimately, puts in solfa the homeostasis of the body [37]. On the other hand, some authors, relying on the use of food to relieve moments of high anxiety that people have from time to time, raise the consideration of binge eating disorder as a subtype of obesity [38]. But the truth is that it is common to find manuals or books on the ED in which obesity is treated without making it abundantly clear that this is not a mental disorder [39].

The truth is also that the figures that reach overweight and obesity in countries such as the United States, Spain, etc. can be worrying. The Spanish Ministry of Health, Social Services and Equality reports that "the prevalence of obesity in adults reached 16.91% in 2014, maintaining the high levels achieved in 2009 (16.0%) and 2011 (17.03%), in the upward line of the last 25 years [40] and now slightly higher in men than in women. According to the same ministry, since 1987 obesity in the case of women has doubled, and in the case of men the problem is even greater, since it rose from 7 to 17%,1%; maintaining the prevalence of overweight in these same years stable around 32–35%. In 2014, if the figures for overweight and obesity were added, the figure was 52.7% (men 60.7 and women 44.7%).

Fat in medicine, according to Fischler [1], is going to be considered a useless substance, so much so that it is not considered worthy of research on it. This point would be reached through the translation of a series of social processes into the symbolic realm that dominates medicine. The social processes in which lipophobic arises would be [1]: the role of technology in today's society, the division of sexual roles and the modern conception of the individual and the relationships that the latter maintains with the collective.

This author [1] points out the decisive role of American insurance companies in the resignation of obesity as a risk factor for health. In 1890 it is noted that fatness reduces people's life expectancy, but in 1951 statistical support is given to this observation. Metropolitan Life concluded that "obesity increases mortality very dramatically" [1]. But the problem was that according to Fischler [1] this statistic lacked sufficient methodological rigor: the sample was not representative of the universe; the rigor of the data collection was not desirable (weights were made with clothes and shoes on) etc. On the basis of all this Fischler concludes that:

> *Be that as it may, Metropolitan Life studies served as the basis for a vast campaign of insurance companies to incite the population to lose weight. American doctors, subjected to an intense campaign, easily adopted the conclusions and considered the duty to disseminate them and to advocate widespread weight loss [1].*

From this moment a series of processes occur that affect and increase the phobia to fat [1]:

- The criminalization of sugar: this food is considered bad at all times and places.
- The criminalization of cholesterol: cholesterol is indispensable for the survival of the human being; it is part of the cell membranes and makes certain hormones.
- The social stigma associated with fat.

- The canon of beauty.
- The *juvenilization* of society.
- The criminalization of sugar: this food is considered bad at all times and places.

4. Conclusions

To end with, it can be said that obesity advanced vertiginously from a social situation, a personal characteristic, to be considered a medical problem. The aforementioned medical situation, in turn, would go from being considered a risk factor, to a disease, and even an epidemic of global proportions [26]. Thus, in Western societies come from two processes that intersected in the current standardization of food: the medicalization of food and the moralization of it. This produced the current dietary standardization that comes from criminalizing half of the western population labelling it as obese. From that moment on, all the dietary food imaginary linked obesity to meanings of personal weakness, lack of will of people, etc. Which can cause the typical vicious circle of so-called obesogenic societies to arise. Better not to say: "When prescribing slimming diets, many doctors consider that the carriers of the anomaly -excess fat- are responsible for their dysfunction: if you are obese, it is because you eat a lot or because you do not know or do not want to eat well" [26].

In this way it is necessary to take into account that for the explained it is possible that the stigma effects of some tide to the ED. It should be known whether it affects only the general population or whether it may also affect the perception of professionals of the persons affected by any of the disorders covered by this research.

Author details

Juan José Labora González* and Pablo Soto-Casás
University of Santiago de Compostela, Santiago de Compostela, Spain

*Address all correspondence to: juan.labora@usc.es

References

[1] Fischler C. El (h)omnívoro. El gusto, la cocina y el cuerpo. Barcelona: Anagrama; 1995. p. 416

[2] Goody J. Cocina cuisine y clase: Estudio de sociología comparada. Barcelona: Gedisa; 1995. p. 312

[3] Douglas M. Símbolos naturales (1ª reimp., e. o. 1970). Madrid: Alianza Editorial; 1988. p. 198

[4] Harris M. Bueno para comer. Madrid: Alianza Editorial; 1990. p. 400

[5] Harris M. Antropología Cultural. 8th ed. Madrid: Alianza Editorial; 2006. p. 656

[6] Harris M. Canívales y reyes. 9th ed. Madrid: Alianza Editorial; 2009. p. 368

[7] Mauss M. Sociología y Antropología. Madrid: Tecnos; 1971. p. 431

[8] Herrera P. Del comer al nutrir. La ignorancia ilustrada del comensal moderno. Madrid: Plaza y Valdés; 2010. p. 326

[9] Coveney J. Food, Morals and Meaning. The Pleasure and Anxiety of Eating. 2nd ed. New York: Routledge; 2006. p. 208. DOI: 10.4324/9780203967355

[10] Friedland WH. La Nueva Globalización: el caso de los productos frescos. In: Bonnano A, editor. La Globalización del Sector Agroalimentario Ministerio de Agricultura. Madrid: Alimentación y Medio Ambiente; 1994. pp. 273-309

[11] Ritzer G. La McDonalización de la sociedad: Un análisis de la racionalización en la vida cotidiana. Barcelona: Ariel; 1996. p. 256

[12] Gracia-Arnáiz M. La transformación de la cultura alimentaria. Cambios y permanencias de un contexto urbano. Ministerio de Educación y. Madrid: Cultura; 1997. p. 318

[13] Gracia-Arnáiz M, editor. Somos lo que comemos. Estudios de alimentación y cultura en España. Barcelona: Ariel; 2002. p. 377

[14] Beck U. La sociedad del riesgo. Hacia una nueva modernidad. Barcelona: Paidós; 2013. p. 400

[15] Luhmann N. Sociología del riesgo. 3rd ed. México D.F.: Universidad Iberoamericana; 2006. p. 158

[16] Luhmann N. La sociedad de la sociedad. Barcelona: Herder/Universidad Iberoamericana; 2007. p. 1024

[17] Luhmann N. El concepto de riesgo. In: Beriain J, editor. (Comp.) Las consecuencias perversas de la modernidad. 2nd ed. Barcelona: Anthropos; 2007. p. 288

[18] Fullagar S. Governing women's active leisure: The gendered effects of calculation rationalities within Australian health policy. Critical Public Health. 2003;**13**:47-60. DOI: 10.1080/0958159031000100206

[19] Gracia-Arnáiz M, Comelles JM, editors. No comerás. Narrativas sobre comida, cuerpo y género en el nuevo milenio. Barcelona: Icaria; 2007. p. 288

[20] Toro J. El cuerpo como delito. Anorexia, bulimia, cultura y sociedad. Barcelona: Ariel; 2015. p. 368

[21] Sanders T, Balzagette P. You Don't Have to Diet. New York: Bantam; 1994. p. 192

[22] Moreno Pestaña JL. Moral corporal, trastornos alimentarios y clase social. Madrid: Centro de Investigaciones Sociológicas; 2010. p. 271

[23] Gordon RA. Anorexia y Bulimia. Anatomía de una epidemia social. Barcelona: Ariel; 1994. p. 253

[24] Malson H. The Thin Woman. Feminism, Pos-structuralism and the Social Psychology of Anorexia Nervosa. New York: Routledge; 1998. p. 252

[25] Vigarello G. La metamorfosis de la grasa. Historia de la obesidad. Barcelona: Península; 2011. p. 368

[26] Gracia-Arnáiz M. Comemos lo que somos. Reflexiones sobre cuerpo, género y salud. Barcelona: Icaria; 2015. p. 272

[27] Raich RM, Sánchez Carracedo D, López Guimerà G. Alimentación, modelo estético femenino y medios de comunicación. 2nd ed. Barcelona: Ministerio de Educación y Ciencia/ Universitat Autònoma de Barcelona; 2008. p. 262

[28] Aristóteles. Problemas. Madrid: Gredos; 2004. p. 221

[29] Gil J. 300 historias de palabras. Cómo nacen y llegan hasta nosotros las palabras que usamos. Barcelona: Círculo de lectores; 2005. p. 360

[30] Phillipe B. El genio y la locura. Barcelona: Ediciones B; 1998. p. 250

[31] Siaud-Facchin J. ¿Demasiado inteligente para ser feliz? Las dificultades del adulto superdotado en la vida cotidiana. 4th ed. Barcelona: Paidós; 2017. p. 304

[32] Pérez Álvarez M. Las raíces de la psicopatología moderna. La melancolía y la esquizofrenia. Madrid: Pirámide; 2012. p. 264

[33] Lama MX. Rosalía de Castro. Cantos de independencia e liberdade (1837-1863). Vigo: Galaxia; 2017. p. 380

[34] Appignanesi L. Mad, Bad and Sad. A History of Women and the Mind Doctors from 1800 to the Present. 2nd ed. London: Virago Press; 2009. p. 554

[35] Chesler P. Women & Madness. New York: Avon; 1972. p. 432

[36] Ussher J. Women's madness. Misogyny or mental illness? Cornwall: Harvester Wheatsheaf; 1991. p. 341

[37] Devlin MJ. Is there place for obesity in DSM-V? International Journal of Eating Disorders. 2007;**40**:83-88. DOI: 10.1002/eat.20430

[38] Devlin MJ, Goldfein JA, Dobrow I. What is this thing called BED? Current status of binge eating disorder nosology? International Journal of Eating Disorders. 2003;**34**:2-18. DOI: 10.1002/eat.10201

[39] Bruch H. Eating Disorders, Obesity, Anorexia Nervosa and the Person Within. New York: BasicBooks, 1973

[40] Encuesta Europea de Salud en España 1987-2014 [Internet]. 2014. Available from: https://www.fen.org.es/storage/app/media/imgPublicaciones/31122015162026.pdf. [Accessed: September 5, 2022]

Chapter 2

Disordered Eating amongst Adolescents

Farzaneh Saeedzadeh Sardahaee

Abstract

Eating disorder, "a persistent disturbance in eating and its related behaviors" affects both "food consumption and its absorption", and the overall physical and mental wellbeing of affected individuals. ED is reported worldwide, across gender, ethnical, racial, and socioeconomic strata. Societal emphasis on gender based body-ideals puts extra pressure on adolescents to achieve or maintain unattainable weigh or body shapes, at the cost of them becoming unwell. ED has a complex etiology where an interplay between genetics and environment brings about the onset of symptoms as early as prepubertal years. With their fluctuating and chronic nature, ED may affect perception, emotions, cognition, and behavior. The interface between ED, overeating and obesity, as well as the recent surge in reported cases of ED during Corona pandemic, has focused much attention on eating pathology amongst adolescents. Many adolescents (particularly boys) specially in a prodromal phases of ED, do not yet meet diagnostic thresholds for ED and hence do not receive timely or appropriate professional help. In the current chapter, we aim to 1- address the issues surrounding early recognition of ED symptoms in adolescents under a general umbrella term, "Disordered Eating", and 2- highlight the importance of societal influence on vulnerable individuals.

Keywords: eating disorder, disordered eating, adolescents, suicidal ideation, mental distress, body ideal, body size overestimation, genetic risk score

1. Introduction

Eating is an integral part of multifaceted human survival behavior, but its importance reaches far beyond human physiological necessities. Eating has helped shape human culture throughout history, by the way of food gathering, its preparation or consumption, as well as through its many symbolic attributes, as evident in fasting, either through spiritual rituals or forced by natural forces such as famine [1]. Some historical accounts of fasting practices date back a few centuries, of which the infamous case of Saint Catherine of Siena, would be considered as eating pathology in more modern times [1, 2].

Overweight and obesity have been known phenomena since prehistoric times [3]. Cases of overeating and consequent purging of food (bulimia) amongst the wealthy are recorded as far back in time as the Middle Ages. Scientific recognition

 IntechOpen

of bulimic practices as a pathology started in the early 1900s; however, the first published scientific article on this condition emerged decades later, in 1979, when the possible link between periodic bulimia and pathological undereating was speculated [4].

Earlier scientific speculations on a link between hunger, varying patterns of food consumption from undereating to bulimia and overweight on one hand and emotional state on the other hand were based on, amongst other observations, coexisting history of some adverse childhood experiences in many cases [5]. A wealth of scientific evidence has been since collected on the complex link between physical and psychological aspects of eating behavior in both general and clinical contexts.

Parallel to an increase in the prevalence of both overweight/obesity and overeating/undereating in the past few decades, adolescents seem to be increasingly concerned with their food consumption, weight, or body size. Although in the past few decades, genetic studies have provided ample evidence for the link between obesity, undereating, and overeating, the current understanding of this link stops short of fully explaining the exact mechanisms underlying a pathological change in eating, from a natural physiological response to hunger/satiety to a disturbed state that can be defined as a medical condition with possible lifelong consequences. Although many times, such disturbing states reach their peak presentation during adolescence and may cause significant health problems for the affected individuals, they may yet not meet the diagnostic criteria for a clinical diagnosis of eating disorder [6, 7].

Eating disorder (ED), as explained extensively elsewhere in this book, refers to a wide range of disturbances in eating and feeding that may vary in their nature, severity, or frequency over the lifespan. In the "Diagnostic and Statistical Manual of Mental Disorders," fifth edition (DSM-V) [8], eating disorders are defined as conditions "*characterized by a persistent disturbance of eating or eating-related behavior that results in the altered consumption or absorption of food and that significantly impairs physical health or psychological functioning*." DSM-V provides diagnostic criteria for an array of ED subtypes: pica, rumination disorders, avoidant/restrictive food intake disorder, anorexia nervosa (AN), bulimia nervosa (BN), binge-eating disorder, other specified feeding or eating disorder (OSFED), and unspecified feeding and eating disorder.

Prevalence, demographics, etiology, and comorbidities in ED are discussed elsewhere in this book and will not be included here. Instead, in this chapter, the author will try to shift readers' attention from ED to a set of similar presentations under an umbrella term, disordered eating (DE) that due to an array of reasons may go unnoticed by clinicians but is nevertheless associated with several biopsychosocial complications.

As an introduction to the subject, the author will first define DE with special attention paid to its common features with ED, before moving on to give a summarized account on prevalence, comorbidities, and burden of disease in DE, followed by a section on etiology on DE, with focus on the importance of societal weight and body ideals, which together with a digitized modern world with an exponential increase in exposure to images portraying such ideals, seem to have created a healthcare dilemma where individuals are advised to maintain a healthy weight, but repeatedly fail to attain societal body ideals that are not necessarily in line with the definition of healthy weight. Treatment in DE follows the same principles employed in treating ED, which is covered in other book chapters and will not be covered here.

Please note in this chapter, the terms ED and DE are not used interchangeably. The term "eating pathology" is used where the author refers to symptom(s) shared between ED and DE.

2. Definition and diagnosis in disordered eating

Over the lifespan of affected individuals, clinical presentations of ED may greatly fluctuate, for instance from anorexia nervosa (AN) to much milder conditions where a diagnosis of ED would no longer apply [9]. Current classification systems, such as the latest edition of WHO's classification system for mental and behavioral disorders, ICD-11 [10], and DSM-V [8], do not match the observed scope of eating problems and their related traits in general adolescent populations, resulting in a considerable proportion of adolescents with an array of eating problems left out with no treatment available to them [11]. On the other hand, heterogeneity, both within and across different subtypes of ED, makes conducting research on ED more challenging and less generalizable, hence the introduction of the umbrella term, disordered eating [12, 13].

Similar to eating disorders, DE is manifested through symptoms such as individuals' concern about their body weight and shape, excessive or unnecessary use of weight reduction methods such as dieting or exercise, self-induced vomiting, inappropriate use of laxative or diuretic, or in some cases periodic binge eating, under- or overweight [14, 15].

Like eating disorders, DE has been associated with varying factors such as "biological" (BMI, puberty), "sociocultural" (socioeconomic status and exposure to media pressure), and "psychological" (early life adverse events, concerns about the body image, self-esteem, and negative affect) [16]. Interestingly, subthreshold symptom constellations observed in DE are associated with similar levels of functional impairment and emotional distress seen in ED [17, 18]. Recognition of impaired function in adolescents with DE is important since, many times, what brings a person to a clinician is their lack of function and not the mere presence or absence of certain symptoms directly taken from medical textbooks.

In clinical settings, the diagnosis of ED is made based on comprehensive clinical interviews and tests, which is a usually lengthy process that requires good training [19, 20]. Self-reported questionnaires [21] are used with the advantage of being quicker and easier to administer than semi-structured diagnostic clinical interviews [19, 22]. One other advantage of self-reported questionnaires is their more accurate reporting of symptoms, such as binge eating, when compared to clinical interviews [19]. Validation studies of self-reported questionnaires in adolescents have shown mixed results, and they are rendered less suitable for screening of eating pathology in overweight adolescents [22, 23].

Attempts have been previously made at making a more robust identification of DE by researchers [11, 22], by using standard screening tools available for ED [23, 24]. These tools are developed on the basis of observations of individuals with more severe presentations than those observed in general populations [25], and they neither seem to have sufficient reliability in the identification of earlier manifestations of ED nor are they fully suitable for the detection of disordered eating [25]. Generally, diagnostic thresholds for DE are either set lower than that for ED, or only a subset of ED symptoms are included in the screening process.

It is important to point out that currently, neither the definition nor identification of DE is fully agreed upon by the scientific community. The author is of the opinion that further identification of more reliable and validated screening tools for DE is important considering that 1 – prevalence of DE is higher than ED [13, 16, 26–28]; 2 – shared symptomatology between ED and DE makes studying the symptoms on their own of value and relevance to a wider group of individuals, independent of their diagnoses; and 3 – a sound understanding of factors attributing to the emergence of symptoms in DE seems pertinent for their prevention. Furthermore, given time, a proportion of adolescents with DE may evolve eating disorders, which makes the development of reliable identification tools for early detection of DE even more important [29].

3. Prevalence and demography in disordered eating

As mentioned earlier, ED and DE have a set of shared symptoms. Previous studies have shown that these symptoms seem to occur worldwide and across many ethnical, racial, and socioeconomic strata [30–32]. Prevalence of these symptoms is reportedly higher than that of clinically diagnosed cases of EDs [31, 33, 34]. Binge eating, purging, and dieting are present across adolescence and adulthood [26, 35–37]. Compared to extreme weight loss or fasting in adolescents that are more commonly flagged up to healthcare services, some prevalent and potentially harmful symptoms such as frequent binge eating and purging may go unreported and hence untreated [16], inadvertently also in populations with DE.

Existing scientific literature has shown that only a small proportion of individuals with ED come to the clinicians' attention [38, 39] partly due to the vigorous application of current diagnostic criteria for ED [39, 40]. On the other hand, the validity of many epidemiological studies on ED has been scrutinized by the scientific community due to their selection bias for younger and fit female populations [38]. This makes research findings derived from clinical populations with ED less generalizable to the general population where targeted preventive methods are meant to be applied [38]. For similar reasons, DE in male adolescents is still understudied [41, 42], hence it is important to have a fresh look at symptoms in a population representing samples, rather than a sole focus on groups with evident clinical diagnoses of ED that have female over-representation.

Although compared to eating disorders, DE is generally milder in its symptomatology, it is more common amongst adolescents than ED [13, 16, 26–28, 43], especially amongst adolescents with higher BMI [44], making DE easier to identify and research in population-based studies.

Similar to ED [19], the symptom constellation in DE may vary based on gender [11]. Both ED and DE are generally more common in females than males [16, 26, 43], but one needs to also bear in mind that 25–30% of preadolescents who attend special ED clinics in Australia and UK are younger males [16, 26]. Moreover, prevalence of binge eating disorder, a subtype of ED with overlapping symptoms with DE, is equal in females and males [45].

4. Comorbidities and burden of disease

The burden of disease in eating pathology remains relatively high since it is associated with poor physical, poorer social relationships and quality of life, lower productivity, higher rates of substance use, anxiety, and depression, as well as increased self-harming behavior, suicidal ideation, suicidal attempts, suicide, and higher mortality [46–53]. Adolescents with overweight, obesity, or those who are unhappy with their weight or shape also show an increase in mental distress. These incremental risks were observed independent of sex, age, BMI, and socioeconomic status, but adolescent boys with DE showed a stronger vulnerability to mental distress [11, 43].

Studies of temporal trends in the burden of disease have shown a considerable increase in the prevalence of binge eating and extreme dieting. Current scientific literature points at a considerable proportion of youth in the USA and Canada reporting high levels of functional impairment due to their attitudes toward eating [7, 27, 38].

Eating pathology may be associated with poor concentration and decision making, as well as with rigidity in thoughts, hence may reducing individuals' mental capacity to recognize their problems or consent to necessary treatments [16]. Lack of timely and effective interventions for EDs can have devastating effects on the lives of sufferers, their families, and wider society. Early detection and timely intervention for eating pathology are vital considering the early age of onset, which is reportedly as low as 10 years old [54], and their possible debilitating effects on the physical and mental wellbeing that can pave the way for a range of unwanted long-term effects. Previous research suggests that increasing treatment coverage could substantially reduce ED-related mortality [32].

5. Etiology in disordered eating

Much of what is known about etiology in DE stems from studies done on symptoms of ED, as previously discussed in this book. The etiology of DE has been difficult to study partially due to its fluctuating and chronic course, and in parts because of its several biopsychosocial determinants. The issues surrounding etiological studies in DE are further complicated by the lack of consensus as how to define DE or classify its subtypes.

The symptom constellation in DE constitutes a range of areas; such as altered perception of weight or body size, negative emotion, changed cognition and behavior such as purging, dieting, extreme or unnecessary exercise, use of diuretics or anabolic steroids as seen in binge eating [8]. Human perception, emotion, cognition, and behavior are shaped and governed by a set of mechanisms that are themselves regulated by the combined effects of genetic and environmental factors, as well as by epigenetics [55–57]. The following subsections briefly look at these factors amongst adolescents with DE, before moving on to expand on the body ideals.

5.1 Genetic factors associated with disordered eating

Identification of heritable patterns in developing DE is important for designing interventions that can detect or modify DE presentations in affected persons, some of whom may develop ED later on in life or see similar presentations in their offspring.

There is a sound scientific ground for generating hypotheses on whether eating pathology, be it a part of ED or DE, shares biopsychosocial determinants with other prevalent public health issues, such as overweight/obesity. Abnormal weight and DE seem to share more than just their phenotypic traits. Family, twin, and adoption studies provide some evidence in favor of a set of common predisposing factors that regulate satiety, appetite, and reward systems in the human brain in both eating pathology and under- or overweight [58–66], for example, through the involvement of dopaminergic and opioid neurotransmitters [67]. A notable observation is the shared genetic susceptibility (FTO, MC4R, BDNF [63, 64], and OPRD1 [28, 60, 65]) between obesity and mechanisms underlying eating pathology. Synaptic plasticity and glutamate receptor activity are pathways that respond to the changes in feeding pattern, such as fasting. Interestingly, these pathways seem to be regulated by obesity-related molecules such as BDNF and MC4R [63, 68–71].

Inheritance studies on subtypes of ED, such as anorexia nervosa, have not identified a single gene with a large effect [72–76]. When no single genetic marker shows a significant effect on the existence of a trait, genetic risk scores (GRSs) have been instead used to study a possible additive effect of several genes on that trait [77]. GRSs have been useful in the identification of shared underlying mechanisms between eating behavior, obesity, ED [78, 79], and satiety [80]. Likewise, GRSs have been used in studying inheritance amongst sex-stratified populations of adolescents with DE [11] where results showed an association between obesity-related genes and DE, as well as observing sex-specific differences in how genes seem to associate with DE symptoms. However, in the absence of a clearer classification of DE symptoms and larger genetic studies, drawing further conclusions on this matter seems premature. Whether these risk factors aggregate in families of individuals with DE is not yet fully understood and needs further research.

5.2 Other factors associated with disordered eating

Investigating the collective effect of biopsychosocial factors in DE at the adolescent age is important since it can help identify individuals at higher risk for developing negative long-term health consequences of eating pathology.

5.2.1 Psychiatric comorbidities

There are reports on a link between negative emotion and regulatory systems involved in food intake [61]. Comorbidity between eating pathology and a wide range of mental disorders, such as anxiety, depression, substance misuse, and personality disorders, is well documented [81–88]. Early life adversities, such as childhood neglect and physical and sexual abuse, have significantly higher prevalence amongst adolescents with eating pathology [35].

5.2.2 Overweight and obesity

Obesity is recognized as a major health problem across the world, also amongst adolescents [89, 90]. In the past few decades, human lifestyle, eating habits, and physical activity together with a subsequent imbalance between food consumption and energy expenditure have undergone major changes [91]. Overweight and obesity have overarching unwanted, yet preventable consequences for both physical and mental health across the lifespan [92]. Like ED and DE, abnormal weight can impair both physical and mental health [92, 93].

The association between weight status, eating pathology and other psychiatric disorders is complex. Both unhealthy weight change and ED are, as shown in animal models, associated with some degree of altered food consumption or absorption [94]. On the other hand, change in eating style has been associated with being overweight or obese, ED, and depressed mood, pointing to the possible association between eating pathology and psychiatric disorders [95]. Moreover, both abnormal weight and ED have a higher prevalence of clinical depression [96, 97], anxiety [98, 99], bipolar affective disorder [100, 101], and substance use disorders [102, 103]. Interestingly, some weight-loss treatment regimens are also known to help improve psychosocial outcomes in obese children with disordered eating [104, 105]. A recent systematic review has shown that the link between obesity and ED is stronger than the link between obesity and depression, anxiety, or substance use disorder [106].

Overweight and obesity were more prevalent in adolescents with DE who show patterns of uncontrolled appetite/overeating compared to those who have poor appetite/undereating. Underweight seems to be more prevalent in adolescents with DE and poor appetite/undereating compared to those who show uncontrolled appetite/overeating [11].

However, it is interesting that despite ample scientific evidence for a close link between abnormal weight and eating pathology, having abnormal weight is not a necessary diagnostic criterion for any ED, or for that matter DE, other than in anorexia nervosa (AN). Neither it is necessary for an individual with abnormal weight to have suffered from any form of DE.

National percentile growth charts show the spread of distribution of weight by height, weight by age, and height by age in a given population of a certain age, gender, and race [107] and are widely used as an indicator of physical development and health from infancy throughout adolescence. Body mass index (BMI), another measure of weight status, has also been used to categorize individuals into underweight, normal weight, overweight, or obese groups [108]. BMI, as originally called Quetelet's Index (QI) [109], is a value derived by quantification of the proportion of mass to height in each individual and is calculated by dividing the body weight in kilograms to the square of the body height in meters (kg/m^2). Use of BMI as an indicator for eating pathology can be particularly misleading amongst adolescent males who may, due to higher muscular volumes and intake of certain supplementary nutrients, have normal BMI even in more debilitating instances of eating pathology.

5.2.3 Societal body ideals

It is also vital to study disordered eating in the context of increasingly more appearance-focused societies, keeping in mind the possible negative effects of unattainable societal body ideals on younger individuals during their formative adolescent years. Societal emphasis on physical appearance may put pressure on adolescents to attain or maintain a certain body type, the so-called body ideals. Many adolescents try to achieve their body ideals by restricting the frequency or content of what they eat, or by vigorous physical exercise, which at times comes at the cost of them neglecting their other needs. Societal stigma about having an eating pathology may prevent adolescents from reporting their problems [110]. It is difficult to identify and costly to treat eating pathology, in part due to a lack of subjective insight into ill-fated consequences of unreported or untreated eating pathology [110, 111].

Body image, a subjective perception of the human body, is a complex construct based on comparisons made between the perception of an individual's body size or shape to that of others. "Size," the magnitude or dimension of a thing, is determined by comparisons drawn between various objects on their magnitude of a quantity, such as mass and length, which could then be expressed either relative to a measuring unit or by assigning adjectives such as smaller/bigger or heavier/smaller.

Mass, weight, or length are separate concepts. In physics, mass is loosely referred to by the amount of "matter" in any given object. Weight, however, refers to something different and more dynamic than the fixed amount of matter in a mass at any given time. Weight is the force that is "experienced" by an object due to gravity. Hence, body image may be considered both "relative" and "subjective," as it may also be dynamic and seen as "amenable to change" [112]. However, human body image seems to be a more complex concept than only a mental picture of dimensions, but rather a multifaceted construct made of neurological, psychological, and sociocultural elements [113].

First scientific studies of body image date back to the 1900s and emerging clinical reports of altered body perception after brain injury in the parietal lobe or phantom limb in amputees. Krueger thought of body image as the representation of identity derived from internal and external body experiences [114]. Schilder attempted at defining body image by combining known concepts of the "somatopsyche," postural model of the body, and the more recent Freudian understanding of ego [113]. In his book, "The Image and Appearance of the Human Body," Schilder suggested that body image plays a fundamental role in individuals' relation to themselves, to their fellow human beings, and to the world around them [113].

Body image is dynamic and may change with individuals' age, mood, or even type of clothing. People with the same body size might have different body weights due to differences in their body composition or muscular and bone density [56, 115]. Discrepancy between subjective body image and actual body size is common in the general population and is a shared feature in many conditions, such as body dysmorphic disorder, obesity, or some types of ED [6]. Besides, human perception is not just a passive reception of sensory information but is also formed by the percipient's cognition that in turn is dependent upon learning, memory, and attention, as well as on pre-learned concepts or expectations (body ideals) [116, 117].

Mismatch between body image and body ideals may lead to unnecessary concern. Concerns about weight or body size are present in various subtypes of ED [8]. Being dissatisfied with one's body is known to associate with changes in affect, lower self-esteem, and social dysfunction [118]. Interestingly, weight underestimation has been associated with less symptoms of anxiety/depression in both adulthood [119] and preadulthood [120].

Individuals with weight or body size concerns may unnecessarily resort to ways to change their appearances, such as dieting or exercise. Many dieting regimes are advertised and endorsed by the society as effective ways to "look better," despite, at times, their questionable effectivity. Subjective body dissatisfaction arising from discrepancy between one's body image and body ideals, combined with individuals' perceived inability to change their appearance by dieting or exercise, can cause or worsen mental distress and may lead to other negative health outcomes [121].

Considering selective mechanisms such as "attention" also influence human perception [122], one can postulate whether focus on body size, may by itself, shape as well as distort, individuals' body image, alter their behavior (dieting) or even mental state.

Societal body ideals are gender based [119], which makes it interesting to examine gender differences in exhibiting weight concern, body size perception, and mental distress. It is also tempting to postulate that pre-learned expectations of how a body should look like (body ideals), as represented in visual clues available through social media or fashion industry, can hypothetically affect individuals' body image.

Association studies between adolescents' BMI, weight concern, body size perception, or dieting and their mental health have provided some answers to these questions [43]. For example, having weight concern has been associated with increased odds of mental distress amongst adolescent boys and girls, to a greater degree than actually being overweight/obese. Similarly, body size overestimation at adolescence has shown a greater impact on mental distress amongst adolescents, than weight concern. Male adolescents who overestimate their body size were shown to be at particularly high risk for having mental distress, compared to their female counterparts [43].

DOI: http://dx.doi.org/10.5772/intechopen.107302

6. Conclusions

Disordered eating at adolescence is prevalent but understudied. The importance of research in the field, especially amongst adolescent males, cannot be overemphasized as these adolescents may suffer from both physical and psychiatric consequences of their eating pathology.

The underlying molecular biology in disordered eating is still understudied. Genetics cannot fully explain the variation in the formation, severity, and course of disordered eating amongst individuals with similar faulty genes. The use of the polygenetic risk score (PRS) in future genetic studies may help quantify the actual genetic risk in each individual carrying these faulty genes.

Furthermore, variation in individuals' response to standard medical and non-medical interventions for disorders of feeding and eating underscores the importance of taking a holistic approach to studying the combined effect of genetic and environmental factors. Epigenetic studies can shed light on resilience factors that may protect young adolescents against developing disordered eating in the first place. Besides, by identification of environmental factors that act as trigger for developing disordered eating, epigenetic studies can help introduce timely and appropriate preventive measures in young adolescents.

Likewise, developing novel intervention methods that can address both disordered eating and comorbid disorders requires studying these disorders together. However, relative lower prevalence of some forms of ED would translate to fewer potential research participants from clinical settings where treatment is sanctioned for more severely affected individuals. Whilst international consortia and multicenter studies are useful ways to overcome this problem, they may introduce other issues such as heterogeneity in study population that may potentially affect study findings and their interpretations.

Future longitudinal studies that focus on traits rather than clinical diagnoses may offer a methodological solution by increasing the number of research participants in any given category of ED symptoms and traits. Findings of population-based studies are more generalizable to nonclinical populations and may better help design preventive measures that fit young adolescents who have not yet reached the disease threshold.

Scientific literature provides evidence for the relative importance of subjective weight concern, rather than being overweight/obese in adolescent mental health. Body size overestimation is associated with mental distress, especially in boys. Body size overestimation and weight concern seemed associated with mental distress, the former playing a greater part. Body size overestimation may be related to increasingly unattainable societal body ideals. Lack of effective weight control methods combined with easy access to relatively cheaper fattening food and overeating has led to an increase in overweight as well as dissatisfaction with own body. The use of compensatory weight reduction behaviors, such as dieting, extreme exercise, and use of anabolic steroids, has also been on the rise amongst adolescents. A change of societal body ideals to a set of more attainable and population representative size or shape may help prevent negative consequences of unnecessary weight concerns or dieting.

Despite showing higher mental health vulnerabilities, male adolescents with DE are an overlooked group. A more thorough examination of DE traits in formative adolescent age is necessary for the early identification of vulnerable adolescents.

Author details

Farzaneh Saeedzadeh Sardahaee[1,2]

1 National Unit for Mandatory Care, St. Olav University Hospital, Trondheim, Norway

2 Center for Research and Education in Security, Prison and Forensic Psychiatry, St. Olav University Hospital, Trondheim, Norway

*Address all correspondence to: farzaneh.sardahaee@googlemail.com

References

[1] Sukkar I, Gagan M, Kealy-Bateman W. The 14th century religious women Margery Kempe and Catherine of Siena can still teach us lessons about eating disorders today. Journal of Eating Disorders. 2017;**5**:23

[2] Galassi FM, Bender N, Habicht ME, et al. Catherine of Siena (1347-1380 AD): One of the earliest historic cases of altered gustatory perception in anorexia mirabilis. Neurological Sciences. 2018;**39**:939-940

[3] Kopelman P. Health risks associated with overweight and obesity. Obesity Reviews. 2007;**8**(Suppl. 1):13-17

[4] Russell G. Bulimia nervosa: an ominous variant of anorexia nervosa. Psychological Medicine. 1979;**9**(3):429-448

[5] Bruch H. Eating Disorders: Obesity, Anorexia Nervosa, and the Person within. New York: Basic Books. 1973

[6] Abebe DS, Lien L, von Soest T. The development of bulimic symptoms from adolescence to young adulthood in females and males: A population-based longitudinal cohort study. The International Journal of Eating Disorders. 2012;**45**(6):737-745

[7] Stice E, Marti CN, Rohde P. Prevalence, incidence, impairment, and course of the proposed DSM-5 eating disorder diagnoses in an 8-year prospective community study of young women. Journal of Abnormal Psychology. 2013;**122**(2):445-457

[8] Association AP. Diagnostic and Statistical Manual of Mental Disorders. Fifth ed. Washington, DC: Feeding and Eating Disorders; 2013

[9] Arlington V. Feed & Eating Disorders in Diagnostic and Statistical Manual of Mental Disorders. 5th ed. Washington, DC: American Psychiatric Association; 2013

[10] WHO. ICD-11: International Classification of Diseases (11th Revision). Geneva, Switzerland: World Health Organization. 2019

[11] Sardahaee FS, Holmen TL, Micali N, Kvaloy K. Effects of single genetic variants and polygenic obesity risk scores on disordered eating in adolescents - the HUNT study. Appetite. 2017;**118**:8-16

[12] Lewinsohn PM, Striegel-Moore RH, Seeley JR. Epidemiology and natural course of eating disorders in young women from adolescence to young adulthood. Journal of the American Academy of Child and Adolescent Psychiatry. 2000;**39**(10):1284-1292

[13] Treasure J, Claudino AM, Zucker N. Eating disorders. Lancet (London, England). 2010;**375**(9714):583-593

[14] Ricciardelli LA, McCabe MP. A biopsychosocial model of disordered eating and the pursuit of muscularity in adolescent boys. Psychological Bulletin. 2004;**130**(2):179-205

[15] Toni G, Berioli MG, Cerquiglini L, Ceccarini G, Grohmann U, Principi N, et al. Eating disorders and disordered eating symptoms in adolescents with type 1 diabetes. Nutrients. 2017;**9**(8):906

[16] Bould H, Newbegin C, Stewart A, Stein A, Fazel M. Eating disorders in children and young people. BMJ (Clinical research ed). 2017;**359**:j5245

[17] Keel PK, Brown TA, Holm-Denoma J, Bodell LP. Comparison of DSM-IV versus

proposed DSM-5 diagnostic criteria for eating disorders: Reduction of eating disorder not otherwise specified and validity. The International Journal of Eating Disorders. 2011;**44**(6):553-560

[18] Stice E, Becker CB, Yokum S. Eating disorder prevention: Current evidence-base and future directions. The International Journal of Eating Disorders. 2013;**46**(5):478-485

[19] Bryant-Waugh RJ, Cooper PJ, Taylor CL, Lask BD. The use of the eating disorder examination with children: A pilot study. The International Journal of Eating Disorders. 1996;**19**(4):391-397

[20] Crist W, Napier-Phillips A. Mealtime behaviors of young children: A comparison of normative and clinical data. Journal of Developmental and Behavioral Pediatrics. 2001;**22**(5):279-286

[21] Carey M, Kupeli N, Knight R, Troop NA, Jenkinson PM, Preston C. Eating disorder examination questionnaire (EDE-Q): Norms and psychometric properties in U.K. females and males. Psychological Assessment. 2019;**31**(7):839-850

[22] Bjornelv S. Eating- and Weight Problems in Adolescents, the Young-HUNT Study. Norway: Norwegian University of Science and Technology (NTNU); 2009

[23] Kraemer HC. Evaluating medical tests - objective and quantitative guidelines. SAGE Publications. 1992:1243

[24] Mairs R, Nicholls D. Assessment and treatment of eating disorders in children and adolescents. Archives of Disease in Childhood. 2016;**101**(12):1168-1175

[25] Offord DR, Kraemer HC, Kazdin AE, Jensen PS, Harrington R. Lowering the burden of suffering from child psychiatric disorder: Trade-offs among clinical, targeted, and universal interventions. Journal of the American Academy of Child and Adolescent Psychiatry. 1998;**37**(7):686-694

[26] Smink FR, van Hoeken D, Oldehinkel AJ, Hoek HW. Prevalence and severity of DSM-5 eating disorders in a community cohort of adolescents. The International journal of eating disorders. 2014;**47**(6):610-619

[27] Culbert KM, Burt SA, McGue M, Iacono WG, Klump KL. Puberty and the genetic diathesis of disordered eating attitudes and behaviors. Journal of Abnormal Psychology. 2009;**118**(4):788-796

[28] Micali N, Field AE, Treasure JL, Evans DM. Are obesity risk genes associated with binge eating in adolescence? Obesity (Silver Spring). 2015;**23**(8):1729-1736

[29] Jacobi C, Hayward C, de Zwaan M, Kraemer HC, Agras WS. Coming to terms with risk factors for eating disorders: Application of risk terminology and suggestions for a general taxonomy. Psychological Bulletin. 2004;**130**(1):19-65

[30] Mitchison D, Hay P, Slewa-Younan S, Mond J. The changing demographic profile of eating disorder behaviors in the community. BMC Public Health. 2014;**14**:943

[31] Mitchison D, Hay P, Slewa-Younan S, Mond J. Time trends in population prevalence of eating disorder behaviors and their relationship to quality of life. PLoS One. 2012;**7**(11):e48450

[32] Schaumberg K, Welch E, Breithaupt L, Hubel C, Baker JH, Munn-Chernoff MA, et al. The science behind the academy for eating Disorders' nine truths about eating disorders. European Eating Disorders Review. 2017;**25**(6):432-450

[33] Miller MN, Pumariega AJ. Culture and eating disorders: A historical and cross-cultural review. Psychiatry. 2001;**64**(2):93-110

[34] Wadden TA, Foster GD, Sarwer DB, Anderson DA, Gladis M, Sanderson RS, et al. Dieting and the development of eating disorders in obese women: Results of a randomized controlled trial. The American Journal of Clinical Nutrition. 2004;**80**(3):560-568

[35] Hay PJ, Mond J, Buttner P, Darby A. Eating disorder behaviors are increasing: Findings from two sequential community surveys in South Australia. PLoS One. 2008;**3**(2):e1541

[36] Ward ZJ, Rodriguez P, Wright DR, Austin SB, Long MW. Estimation of eating disorders prevalence by age and associations with mortality in a simulated nationally representative US cohort. JAMA Network Open. 2019;**2**(10):e1912925

[37] Smink FR, van Hoeken D, Hoek HW. Epidemiology, course, and outcome of eating disorders. Current Opinion in Psychiatry. 2013;**26**(6):543-548

[38] Jones JM, Bennett S, Olmsted MP, Lawson ML, Rodin G. Disordered eating attitudes and behaviours in teenaged girls: A school-based study. CMAJ. 2001;**165**(5):547-552

[39] Keski-Rahkonen A, Mustelin L. Epidemiology of eating disorders in Europe: Prevalence, incidence, comorbidity, course, consequences, and risk factors. Current Opinion in Psychiatry. 2016;**29**(6):340-345

[40] Susser E, Patel V. Psychiatric epidemiology and global mental health: Joining forces. International Journal of Epidemiology. 2014;**43**(2):287-293

[41] Sweeting H, Walker L, MacLean A, Patterson C, Raisanen U, Hunt K. Prevalence of eating disorders in males: A review of rates reported in academic research and UK mass media. International Journal of Men's Health. 2015;**14**(2):10

[42] Murray SB, Nagata JM, Griffiths S, Calzo JP, Brown TA, Mitchison D, et al. The enigma of male eating disorders: A critical review and synthesis. Clinical Psychology Review. 2017;**57**:1-11

[43] Saeedzadeh Sardahaee F, Kvaloy K. Cross-sectional study of BMI, weight concern, body size perception, dieting and mental distress in adolescents: The HUNT study. BMJ Open. 2022;**12**(4):e045962

[44] Striegel-Moore RH, Franko DL. Epidemiology of binge eating disorder. The International Journal of Eating Disorders. 2003;**34**(Suppl):S19-S29

[45] Mustelin L, Bulik CM, Kaprio J, Keski-Rahkonen A. Prevalence and correlates of binge eating disorder related features in the community. Appetite. 2017;**109**:165-171

[46] Stuhldreher N, Konnopka A, Wild B, Herzog W, Zipfel S, Lowe B, et al. Cost-of-illness studies and cost-effectiveness analyses in eating disorders: A systematic review. The International Journal of Eating Disorders. 2012;**45**(4):476-491

[47] Striegel Weissman R, Rosselli F. Reducing the burden of suffering from eating disorders: Unmet treatment needs, cost of illness, and the quest for cost-effectiveness. Behaviour Research and Therapy. 2017;**88**:49-64

[48] Lal M, Abraham S. Adolescent development and eating disorder related quality of life in Indian females. Eating and Weight Disorders: EWD. 2011;**16**(1):e56-e60

[49] Perez M, Warren CS. The relationship between quality of life, binge-eating disorder, and obesity status in an ethnically diverse sample. Obesity (Silver Spring). 2012;**20**(4):879-885

[50] Agh T, Kovacs G, Pawaskar M, Supina D, Inotai A, Voko Z. Epidemiology, health-related quality of life and economic burden of binge eating disorder: A systematic literature review. Eating and Weight Disorders: EWD. 2015;**20**(1):1-12

[51] Hay P, Mitchison D, Collado AEL, Gonzalez-Chica DA, Stocks N, Touyz S. Burden and health-related quality of life of eating disorders, including avoidant/restrictive food intake disorder (ARFID), in the Australian population. Journal of Eating Disorders. 2017;**5**:21

[52] Goldstein A, Gvion Y. Socio-demographic and psychological risk factors for suicidal behavior among individuals with anorexia and bulimia nervosa: A systematic review. Journal of Affective Disorders. 2019;**245**:1149-1167

[53] Crow S, Eisenberg ME, Story M, Neumark-Sztainer D. Suicidal behavior in adolescents: Relationship to weight status, weight control behaviors, and body dissatisfaction. The International Journal of Eating Disorders. 2008;**41**(1):82-87

[54] Borges G, Benjet C, Medina-Mora ME, Orozco R, Nock M. Suicide ideation, plan, and attempt in the Mexican adolescent mental health survey. Journal of the American Academy of Child and Adolescent Psychiatry. 2008;**47**(1):41-52

[55] Plomin R, Haworth CM, Davis OS. Common disorders are quantitative traits. Nature Reviews. Genetics. 2009;**10**(12):872-878

[56] Gelernter J. Genetics of complex traits in psychiatry. Biological Psychiatry. 2015;**77**(1):36-42

[57] Zerwas S, Bulik CM. Genetics and epigenetics of eating disorders. Psychiatric Annals. 2011;**41**(11):532-538

[58] Bulik-Sullivan B, Finucane HK, Anttila V, Gusev A, Day FR, Loh PR, et al. An atlas of genetic correlations across human diseases and traits. Nature Genetics. 2015;**47**(11):1236-1241

[59] Kvaloy K, Holmen J, Hveem K, Holmen TL. Genetic effects on longitudinal changes from healthy to adverse weight and metabolic status - the HUNT study. PLoS One. 2015;**10**(10):e0139632

[60] Kvaloy K, Kulle B, Romundstad P, Holmen TL. Sex-specific effects of weight-affecting gene variants in a life course perspective--the HUNT study, Norway. International Journal of Obesity. 2013;**37**(9):1221-1229

[61] Gorwood P, Blanchet-Collet C, Chartrel N, Duclos J, Dechelotte P, Hanachi M, et al. New insights in anorexia nervosa. Frontiers in Neuroscience. 2016;**10**:256

[62] Peckmezian T, Hay P. A systematic review and narrative synthesis of interventions for uncomplicated obesity: Weight loss, well-being and impact on eating disorders. Journal of Eating Disorders. 2017;**5**:15

[63] Locke AE, Kahali B, Berndt SI, Justice AE, Pers TH, Day FR, et al. Genetic studies of body mass index yield new insights for obesity biology. Nature. 2015;**518**(7538):197-206

[64] Speliotes EK, Willer CJ, Berndt SI, Monda KL, Thorleifsson G, Jackson AU, et al. Association analyses of 249,796 individuals reveal 18 new loci associated with body mass index. Nature Genetics. 2010;**42**(11):937-948

[65] Scherag S, Hebebrand J, Hinney A. Eating disorders: The current status of

molecular genetic research. European Child & Adolescent Psychiatry. 2010;**19**(3):211-226

[66] Castellini G, Franzago M, Bagnoli S, Lelli L, Balsamo M, Mancini M, et al. Fat mass and obesity-associated gene (FTO) is associated to eating disorders susceptibility and moderates the expression of psychopathological traits. PLoS One. 2017;**12**(3):e0173560

[67] Kessler RM, Hutson PH, Herman BK, Potenza MN. The neurobiological basis of binge-eating disorder. Neuroscience and Biobehavioral Reviews. 2016;**63**:223-238

[68] Yang Y, Atasoy D, Su HH, Sternson SM. Hunger states switch a flip-flop memory circuit via a synaptic AMPK-dependent positive feedback loop. Cell. 2011;**146**(6):992-1003

[69] Qi Y, Yang Y. Hunger states control the directions of synaptic plasticity via switching cell type-specific subunits of NMDA receptors. The Journal of Neuroscience. 2015;**35**(38):13171-13182

[70] Wu Q, Clark MS, Palmiter RD. Deciphering a neuronal circuit that mediates appetite. Nature. 2012;**483**(7391):594-597

[71] Shen Y, Fu WY, Cheng EY, Fu AK, Ip NY. Melanocortin-4 receptor regulates hippocampal synaptic plasticity through a protein kinase A-dependent mechanism. The Journal of Neuroscience. 2013;**33**(2):464-472

[72] Boraska V, Davis OS, Cherkas LF, Helder SG, Harris J, Krug I, et al. Genome-wide association analysis of eating disorder-related symptoms, behaviors, and personality traits. American Journal of Medical Genetics. Part B, Neuropsychiatric Genetics. 2012;**159B**(7):803-811

[73] Boraska V, Franklin CS, Floyd JA, Thornton LM, Huckins LM, Southam L, et al. A genome-wide association study of anorexia nervosa. Molecular Psychiatry. 2014;**19**(10):1085-1094

[74] Pinheiro AP, Root T, Bulik CM. The genetics of anorexia nervosa: Current findings and future perspectives. International Journal of Child and Adolescent Health. 2009;**2**(2):153-164

[75] Pinheiro AP, Bulik CM, Thornton LM, Sullivan PF, Root TL, Bloss CS, et al. Association study of 182 candidate genes in anorexia nervosa. American Journal of Medical Genetics. Part B, Neuropsychiatric Genetics. 2010;**153B**(5):1070-1080

[76] Root TL, Szatkiewicz JP, Jonassaint CR, Thornton LM, Pinheiro AP, Strober M, et al. Association of candidate genes with phenotypic traits relevant to anorexia nervosa. European Eating Disorders Review. 2011;**19**(6):487-493

[77] Dudbridge F. Power and predictive accuracy of polygenic risk scores. PLoS Genetics. 2013;**9**(3):e1003348

[78] Konttinen H, Llewellyn C, Wardle J, Silventoinen K, Joensuu A, Mannisto S, et al. Appetitive traits as behavioural pathways in genetic susceptibility to obesity: A population-based cross-sectional study. Scientific Reports. 2015;**5**:14726

[79] Steinsbekk S, Belsky D, Guzey IC, Wardle J, Wichstrom L. Polygenic risk, appetite traits, and weight gain in middle childhood: A longitudinal study. JAMA Pediatrics. 2016;**170**(2):e154472

[80] Llewellyn CH, Trzaskowski M, van Jaarsveld CHM, Plomin R, Wardle J. Satiety mechanisms in genetic risk of obesity. JAMA Pediatrics. 2014;**168**(4):338-344

[81] Fernandez-Aranda F, Pinheiro AP, Tozzi F, Thornton LM, Fichter MM, Halmi KA, et al. Symptom profile of major depressive disorder in women with eating disorders. The Australian and New Zealand Journal of Psychiatry. 2007;**41**(1):24-31

[82] Thornton LM, Watson HJ, Jangmo A, Welch E, Wiklund C, von Hausswolff-Juhlin Y, et al. Binge-eating disorder in the Swedish national registers: Somatic comorbidity. The International Journal of Eating Disorders. 2017;**50**(1):58-65

[83] Swinbourne JM, Touyz SW. The co-morbidity of eating disorders and anxiety disorders: A review. European Eating Disorders Review. 2007;**15**(4):253-274

[84] Salbach-Andrae H, Lenz K, Simmendinger N, Klinkowski N, Lehmkuhl U, Pfeiffer E. Psychiatric comorbidities among female adolescents with anorexia nervosa. Child Psychiatry and Human Development. 2008;**39**(3):261-272

[85] Halmi KA, Sunday SR, Klump KL, Strober M, Leckman JF, Fichter M, et al. Obsessions and compulsions in anorexia nervosa subtypes. The International Journal of Eating Disorders. 2003;**33**(3):308-319

[86] Hoffman ER, Gagne DA, Thornton LM, Klump KL, Brandt H, Crawford S, et al. Understanding the association of impulsivity, obsessions, and compulsions with binge eating and purging behaviours in anorexia nervosa. European Eating Disorders Review. 2012;**20**(3):e129-e136

[87] Bulik CM, Klump KL, Thornton L, Kaplan AS, Devlin B, Fichter MM, et al. Alcohol use disorder comorbidity in eating disorders: A multicenter study. The Journal of Clinical Psychiatry. 2004;**65**(7):1000-1006

[88] Krug I, Pinheiro AP, Bulik C, Jimenez-Murcia S, Granero R, Penelo E, et al. Lifetime substance abuse, family history of alcohol abuse/dependence and novelty seeking in eating disorders: Comparison study of eating disorder subgroups. Psychiatry and Clinical Neurosciences. 2009;**63**(1):82-87

[89] Xu S, Xue Y. Pediatric obesity: Causes, symptoms, prevention and treatment. Experimental and Therapeutic Medicine. 2016;**11**(1):15-20

[90] Collaboration NCDRF. Worldwide trends in body-mass index, underweight, overweight, and obesity from 1975 to 2016: A pooled analysis of 2416 population-based measurement studies in 128.9 million children, adolescents, and adults. Lancet (London, England). 2017;**390**(10113):2627-2642

[91] Couzin-Franke J. Tackling America's eating habits, one store at a time. Science. 2012;**337**(6101):1473-1475

[92] Greydanus DE, Agana M, Kamboj MK, Shebrain S, Soares N, Eke R, et al. Pediatric obesity: Current concepts. Disease-a-Month. 2018;**64**(4):98-156

[93] Galvez JF, Bauer IE, Sanches M, Wu HE, Hamilton JE, Mwangi B, et al. Shared clinical associations between obesity and impulsivity in rapid cycling bipolar disorder: A systematic review. Journal of Affective Disorders. 2014;**168**:306-313

[94] Himmerich H, Bentley J, Kan C, Treasure J. Genetic risk factors for eating disorders: An update and insights into pathophysiology. Therapeutic Advances in Psychopharmacology. 2019;**9**:2045125318814734

[95] Paans NPG, Bot M, van Strien T, Brouwer IA, Visser M, Penninx B. Eating styles in major depressive disorder: Results from a large-scale study. Journal of Psychiatric Research. 2018;**97**:38-46

[96] Godart N, Radon L, Curt F, Duclos J, Perdereau F, Lang F, et al. Mood disorders in eating disorder patients: Prevalence and chronology of ONSET. Journal of Affective Disorders. 2015;**185**:115-122

[97] Jantaratnotai N, Mosikanon K, Lee Y, McIntyre RS. The interface of depression and obesity. Obesity Research & Clinical Practice. 2017;**11**(1):1-10

[98] Ulfvebrand S, Birgegard A, Norring C, Hogdahl L, von Hausswolff-Juhlin Y. Psychiatric comorbidity in women and men with eating disorders results from a large clinical database. Psychiatry Research. 2015;**230**(2):294-299

[99] Sagar R, Gupta T. Psychological aspects of obesity in children and adolescents. Indian Journal of Pediatrics. 2018;**85**(7):554-559

[100] McDonald CE, Rossell SL, Phillipou A. The comorbidity of eating disorders in bipolar disorder and associated clinical correlates characterised by emotion dysregulation and impulsivity: A systematic review. Journal of Affective Disorders. 2019;**259**:228-243

[101] Zhao Z, Okusaga OO, Quevedo J, Soares JC, Teixeira AL. The potential association between obesity and bipolar disorder: A meta-analysis. Journal of Affective Disorders. 2016;**202**:120-123

[102] Bahji A, Mazhar MN, Hudson CC, Nadkarni P, MacNeil BA, Hawken E. Prevalence of substance use disorder comorbidity among individuals with eating disorders: A systematic review and meta-analysis. Psychiatry Research. 2019;**273**:58-66

[103] Lanza HI, Grella CE, Chung PJ. Adolescent obesity and future substance use: Incorporating the psychosocial context. Journal of Adolescence. 2015;**45**:20-30

[104] Hayes JF, Fitzsimmons-Craft EE, Karam AM, Jakubiak J, Brown ML, Wilfley DE. Disordered eating attitudes and Behaviors in youth with overweight and obesity: Implications for treatment. Current Obesity Reports. 2018;**7**(3):235-246

[105] Val-Laillet D, Aarts E, Weber B, Ferrari M, Quaresima V, Stoeckel LE, et al. Neuroimaging and neuromodulation approaches to study eating behavior and prevent and treat eating disorders and obesity. NeuroImage: Clinical. 2015;**8**:1-31

[106] Rajan TM, Menon V. Psychiatric disorders and obesity: A review of association studies. Journal of Postgraduate Medicine. 2017;**63**(3):182-190

[107] https://www.cdc.gov/growthcharts/clinical_charts.htm

[108] https://www.cdc.gov/obesity/childhood/defining.html

[109] Garrow JS. Quetelet index as indicator of obesity. Lancet (London, England). 1986;**1**(8491):1219

[110] Ali K, Farrer L, Fassnacht DB, Gulliver A, Bauer S, Griffiths KM. Perceived barriers and facilitators towards help-seeking for eating disorders: A systematic review. The International Journal of Eating Disorders. 2017;**50**(1):9-21

[111] Stein D, Keller S, Ifergan IS, Shilton T, Toledano A, Pelleg MT,

et al. Extreme risk-taking Behaviors in patients with eating disorders. Frontiers in Psychiatry. 2020;**11**:89

[112] Linardon J, Gleeson J, Yap K, Murphy K, Brennan L. Meta-analysis of the effects of third-wave behavioural interventions on disordered eating and body image concerns: Implications for eating disorder prevention. Cognitive Behaviour Therapy. 2019;**48**(1):15-38

[113] Schilder PF. The Image and Appearance of the Human Body. New York: International Universities Press; 1950

[114] Krueger DW. Body Self and Psychological Self: Developmental and Clinical Integration of Disorders of the Self. New York: Brunner/Mazel; 1989

[115] Hubel C, Marzi SJ, Breen G, Bulik CM. Epigenetics in eating disorders: A systematic review. London, Great Britain: Molecular Psychiatry. 2019;**24**(6):901-915

[116] Gregory R. In: Gregory, Zangwill, editors. Perception. 1987. pp. 598-601

[117] Bernstein DA. Essentials of Psychology. Cengage Learning; 2010

[118] Duchesne AP, Dion J, Lalande D, Begin C, Emond C, Lalande G, et al. Body dissatisfaction and psychological distress in adolescents: Is self-esteem a mediator? Journal of Health Psychology. 2017;**22**(12):1563-1569

[119] Kvaloy K, Melhus M, Silviken A, Broderstad AR. Weight underestimation linked to anxiety and depression in a cross-sectional study of overweight individuals in a Sami and non-Sami Norwegian population: The SAMINOR study. BMJ Open. 2019;**9**(11):e031810

[120] Choi E, Choi I. The associations between body dissatisfaction, body figure, self-esteem, and depressed mood in adolescents in the United States and Korea: A moderated mediation analysis. Journal of Adolescence. 2016;**53**:249-259

[121] Irvine KR, McCarty K, McKenzie KJ, Pollet TV, Cornelissen KK, Tovee MJ, et al. Distorted body image influences body schema in individuals with negative bodily attitudes. Neuropsychologia. 2019;**122**:38-50

[122] Kiyonaga A, Scimeca JM, Bliss DP, Whitney D. Serial dependence across perception, attention, and memory. Trends in Cognitive Sciences. 2017;**21**(7):493-497

Chapter 3

Prevalence and Determinants of Obesity in Children in Algeria

Nasreddine Aissaoui, Lamia Hamaizia, Said Khalfa Mokhtar Brika and Ahmed Laamari

Abstract

Our objectives through this paper are multiple: to measure the prevalence of overweight and obesity in children between 5–11 years; highlight the main causes that lead children under 12 years old to become overweight or obese, especially by highlighting the cause and effect relationship between eating disorders "bulimia nervosa" and obesityoverweigh; highlight the risk factors associated with overweight or obese children; and finally, the strategies to be planned and the policies to be applied to curb the phenomenon of obesity in this age group. This is a descriptive and cross-sectional survey which aims to study and analyze a representative sample of children under the age of 12 who attend a municipal swimming pool during the month of July 2018. The sample is made up of 509 children from less than 12 years old; the majority of children are regulars at the municipal swimming pool during the summer located in the department of Constantine, a department in the North-East of Algeria. Overweight affects 14% of children aged 5–11 years old, while moderate obesity affects 4% of children in this age category, frank obesity affects 1% of this age group. The percentage of boys and girls with a BMI3, 4 or 5 are around 13% and 23%, respectively, of the entire sample.

Keywords: overweight and obesity, bulimia nervosa, prevalence of obesity, factors associated with obesity, risk factors for obesity, Algeria

1. Introduction

The prevalence of overweight and obesity has risen at an alarming rate in recent decades, particularly among children and adolescents, becoming one of the greatest public health challenges of the twenty-first century [1, 2]. Childhood and adolescent obesity is a global problem, affecting both developed and low- and middle-income countries, particularly in urban areas [3–5].

In 2019, an estimated 38.2 million children under the age of 5 years were overweight or obese. Once seen as specific problems of high-income countries, overweight and obesity are now on the rise in low- and middle-income countries, particularly in urban settings. In Africa, the number of overweight or obese children has increased by almost 24% since 2000. Almost half of overweight or obese children under 5 years lived in Asia in 2019. More than 340 million children and adolescents aged 5 to 19 years were overweight or obese in 2016 [1].

Overweight and obesity are becoming a serious public health problem; one in two Algerians and one in three Algerian women are overweight [6]. The phenomenon hardly spares children; the tendency to overweight is rather on the rise in a society inclined to a sedentary lifestyle and excessive consumption of fast-food products. Globally, the number of obese children and adolescents aged 5 to 19 years has increased 10-fold over the past four decades. If current trends continue, by 2022 there will be more obese children and adolescents than moderately or severely underweight children [7].

Through a questionnaire, we conducted a survey of children under 12 years old. This survey aims to study and analyze the causes and consequences of overweight or obesity on a sample of children aged 5 to 11 years old.

2. Patients and methods

This was a descriptive cross-sectional study on a representative sample of 509 children between 5 and 11 years old, the survey was conducted during the month of July 2018.

2.1 Study type and population

The study population consisted of 509 children aged 5 to 11 years old, who visit a public swimming pool during the summer holidays. The children are selected by chance, during the 4 weeks of July 2018.

2.2 Study variables

We studied age, sex, height, weight and BMI. The weight, expressed in kilograms, was measured in a lightly dressed, barefoot subject, standing on a SECA digital medical scale (Seca 703 digital column scale with measuring rod, Germany).

BMI was calculated by dividing the weight expressed in kilograms by the square of the height expressed in meters. We used the definition of the International Obesity Task Force/ IOTF [8], which is based on the recommendations of the European Childhood Obesity Group for epidemiological studies of Rolland-Cachera [9].

In 2000, the Childhood Obesity Working Group of the International Obesity Task Force (IOTF), a working group under the aegis of the WHO, developed a new definition of childhood obesity with curves for boys and girls aged 2 to 18 according to the thresholds proposed by Cole et al. [8]. This definition has the specificity of coordinating the characteristics of childhood obesity and adult: it uses the same index (BMI) and refers to the same thresholds. Body mass index (BMI) was calculated by dividing weight by height squared BMI = Weight/Height2 (kg/m2). The International Obesity Task Force (IOTF) proposes 5 BMI groups [9]:

- Group BMI 1 $<$ 20: subjects with a weight deficit;
- Group BMI 2 group between 20 and 25: normal population;

- Group BMI 3 between 25 and 30: overweight;
- Group BMI 4 between 30 and 40: moderate obesity;
- Group BMI 5 > 40: frank obesity (morbid).

In children and adolescents, curves have been developed to take into account the specificity of sex and age.

2.3 Statistical analysis

Using a standardized questionnaire, respecting confidentiality, anonymity and after informing the families. We recorded a few refusals, since we distributed 600 copies of questionnaires, and we recovered only 509, thus a percentage of recovery which is around 84.83%. Most uncollected copies are those of children accompanied by adults who are not their parents. According to the questionnaire, two types of data were collected: information on the parents of the children, and others on the children themselves who were the subject of the study.

Data were analyzed using SPSS 21.0 software. Quantitative variables were represented as mean, standard deviation (SD), 95% confidence interval (95% CI), while qualitative variables were represented as numbers (n) and percentage (%). The p value <0.05 was considered statistically significant and a two-tailed test was used.

3. Results

3.1 Prevalence of overweight and obesity in children by gender

The study sample consists of 509 children aged between 5 and 11 years old, among them 235 males and 274 females. By referring to the thresholds of the International Obesity Task Force/IOTF, we obtained the following results (**Table 1**).

The normal body mass index/BMI2 is around 86.8% in boys and 76.7% in girls. Girls had a significantly higher BMI than boys in all age groups, whether overweight (BMI3) or obese (BMI4 and BMI5). By comparing the two sexes, we can see that the difference between the two sexes in BMI becomes more visible with age. The average weight was 31.61 ± 10.33 kg (i.e. 30.23 ± 10.22 kg for boys and 32.46 ± 11.24 kg for girls) in children aged between 5 and 11 years, that of height was 116.23 ± 15.43 cm (i.e. 115.70 ± 12.68 cm for boys and 118.79 ± 9.68 cm for girls) and that of BMI was 19, 39 ± 4.12 kg/m2 (i.e. 18.96 ± 3.85 kg/m2 for boys and 19.97 ± 4.06 kg/m2 for girls). Overweight affects 14% of children aged between 5 and 11 years old, moderate obesity affects 4% of children and frank obesity affects 1% in this age group. The percentage of boys and girls with a BMI of 3, 4 or 5 is around 13% and 23% respectively of the entire sample. The prevalence of overweight in our study was respectively 14.5% (including 18.2% in girls against 10.2% in boys) and that of obesity was 4.1% (including 5.1% in girls against 3.0% in boys). By comparing the prevalence of overweight between the two sexes, the Pearson test shows quite significant differences in girls than boys, on the other hand the same test shows few differences between the two sexes among those who suffer from obesity (**Table 1**).

Age (years)	Gender	Number	Normal	Overweight	p*	Obesity	p**
5	Boys	31	28	01	0.029	02	0.183
	Girls	32	27	05		00	
	Total	63	55	06		02	
6	Boys	42	35	06	0.383	01	0.091
	Girls	54	45	06		03	
	Total	96	80	12		04	
7	Boys	42	38	04	0.514	00	0.041
	Girls	33	27	03		03	
	Total	75	65	07		03	
8	Boys	35	28	05	0.000	02	0.204
	Girls	61	38	18		05	
	Total	96	66	23		07	
9	Boys	39	32	05	0.683	02	0.088
	Girls	32	25	07		00	
	Total	71	57	12		02	
10	Boys	25	25	00	0.000	00	0.045
	Girls	54	43	08		03	
	Total	79	68	08		03	
11	Boys	21	18	03	0.488	00	0.535
	Girls	08	05	03		00	
	Total	29	23	06		00	
Total	Boys	235	204 (86.8%)	24 (10.2%)	0.000	07 (3.0%)	0.188
	Girls	274	210 (76.7%)	50 (18.2%)		14 (5.1%)	
	Total	509	414 (81.4%)	74 (14.5%)		21(4.1%)	

**p-value: comparison of overweight prevalence between boys and girls.*
***p-value: comparison of prevalence of obesity between boys and girls.*

Table 1.
Prevalence of overweight and obesity in children by gender.

3.2 Factors associated with overweight and obesity according to the study sample

Four main questions have been asked to locate the risk factors responsible for overweight or obesity in children under 12: We have not recorded a relationship between the socioeconomic situation of the family and the BMI of the child; on the other hand, other factors can constitute a major risk for these young people gaining extra pounds (**Table 2**).

We can clearly see that overweight and obesity are indeed present in girls more than in boys; since 68% of those who are overweight (group 1) and 67% of those who suffer from obesity (group 2) are female; i.e. two thirds of those who have

Risk factors	Group 1 (%)	Group 2 (%)	p-value
Boys	32	33	0.480
Girls	68	67	0.510
Family history of overweight and obesity	85	52	0.005
The lack of food culture	53	73	0.019
Non-compliance with recommended daily meals	58	60	0.310
Non-practice of physical activity (sedentary lifestyle)	22	38	0.023

Group 1: those who are overweight (BMI3).
Group 2: those who are obese (BMI4 and BMI5).

Table 2.
Factors associated with overweight and obesity in children.

(BMI3, BMI4 and BMI5). Two out of three of the parents questioned have a medium or high level of education. Weight gain begins early in 85% of children, where the family history is pointed out. We found an absence of a food culture in 53% of the families of children in both groups and an insufficient culture in 32% of the families of children in the two groups. What is worrying in both groups; it is the non-taking of breakfast which is around 58% in children of the two categories, the non-taking of breakfast at home is responsible for the multiple snacks before and after lunch, thus the majority of the children of the two groups have tendency to snack all the time, in other words to have one or more snacks during the day. We noticed that 78% of the children in two groups admitted: never or rarely practicing physical activity during the week outside of school. The majority of "never" or "rarely" answers are those of girls of the two groups, who admit that they never or rarely practice a physical activity outside the school establishment, this percentage is close to 100% among girls aged 10 and 11 years, in the same wake 89% of children admit to spending more than an hour in front of an electronic device for entertainment daily, even during school days.

4. Discussion

In our study, the prevalence of overweight including obesity is 18% in children between 5 and 11 years old, according to the international IOTF thresholds corresponding to BMI4 and 5 in adulthood. We arrived at the following results: 14% of the children in the study sample are overweight, while moderate and frank obesity concerns 4% of this age group. Girls are the most affected by overweight and obesity with 18 and 5% respectively, compared to 10 and 3% for boys. The proportions of overweight and obese children are close to those found in the national literature [4, 5, 10, 11]. However, the situation is changing from 1 year to year, since in 6 years: the prevalence of overweight including obesity is 18% after it was 13.1%; if overweight only affected 10% of children before, now it affects 14%; obesity only affected 3.1% of this age category at the beginning of this decade, now it affects 4% globally according to the most recent study on this age category [4, 5, 12]. The prevalence of overweight including obesity is 24% according to IOTF international thresholds. According to a study conducted in 2013 by the Algerian Nutrition Society (SAN), 13% of adolescents aged 10 to 17 are overweight [6]. Globally, the obesity rate among children continues to rise from 1 year to the next, as this rate has risen from less than 1% in 1975 (i.e. 11 million children), to more than 6%

(i.e. 124 million) in 2016. So these figures show that the number of obese children aged 5 to 19 in the world is multiplied by 10. We must not forget that the number of overweight children is very worrying; we recorded 213 million in 2016. Fortunately, obesity in Algeria is below world averages, but measures must be taken to counter this scourge [1].

The prevalence of overweight is higher in girls than in boys of children between 5 and 11 years old. Thus, girls between the ages of 4 and 11 are 2.08 times more likely to be overweight and twice to become obese, which is consistent with the results of published research [13, 14]. In the present study, we found age to be a factor associated with overweight and obesity. Thus, 14% of children between 5 and 11 years old are overweight, and 4% are obese. Therefore, over the years, weight gain seems inevitable, which is consistent with the results of published research [4, 15]. According to our survey, the birth weight of the child and the BMI of the parents are risk factors for overweight or obesity. Thus, 85% of parents of children who have extra pounds admit that they still have curves. In addition, 52% of children suffering from excess weight have overweight or obese parents; which is consistent with the results of published studies [16–18]. The results of this survey showed that 85% of families ignore or neglect the nutritional content of the meals consumed by their children [19]. In the same vein, 53% of parents of overweight or obese children admit that the nutritional culture of food is not taken into consideration at home, which is consistent with the results of published studies. According to this survey, few children respect the recommended number of meals (i.e. 3–4 meals per day). What is worrying is that 58% of the subjects in the sample do not have breakfast at home in the morning. For those who are overweight or obese, the majority of them take at least two snacks a day, which is consistent with the results of published studies [18, 20, 21]. In the present study, we arrived that 78% of the children do not practice, or rarely, a sports activity outside the school establishment, to tell the truth apart from the 2 hours of physical activity within the school; they have no other sporting activity, which consistent with the results of published studies [4, 18, 22]. Most surprisingly, for those who do not practice any physical activity or rarely outside school, it is the percentage of girls between the ages of 10 and 11 which is close to 100%. This is mainly due to social taboos and the absence of stadiums or sports halls reserved for girls and teenagers. If the non-practice of sporting activity is quite visible, sedentary lifestyle is becoming more and more accentuated among young people. Our results show that 37% of children spend more than 2 hours in front of an electronic entertainment device, so overweight or obese children suffer more from this scourge, who over time become dependent on this kind of leisure.

5. Conclusion

Overweight and obesity have progressed rapidly over the past 5 decades; children are not immune to this phenomenon which affects all age groups, which has become a serious public health problem throughout the world. Algeria is not an exception, since the plural transition that has known this country for the last 4 decades has generated profound changes and bad habits among Algerians, in this case among the children of this country. Since the 1990s, Algeria has experienced an economic transition towards a market economy, and that after more than 30 years of socialism, this economic opening has allowed an abundance of goods on the shelves of supermarkets, among these goods those which do not are not necessarily healthy (sweets, sodas, fast food, etc.). A marked improvement in purchasing power; enabled Algerians to direct their spending towards the impulsive purchase of energy products, fast foods, and fatty meals. Children do not escape this new life, which promotes a sedentary lifestyle and cheap unhealthy meals. The results of our survey confirm the significant increase in overweight and obesity among Algerian children. Our results converge with the majority of results from national and international research, which have sounded the alarm about the dangerousness of the phenomenon and its rapid progression. The responsibility is shared between: parents, schools, media, food industry, etc. In order to fight against the consequences of obesity on our children, in this case chronic diseases, several preventive solutions can be sought: early food education must be taken into consideration in textbooks from primary school; make manufacturers aware of reducing the levels of the three whites (sugar, salt, white flour) in food; encourage homemade meals that protect our dear health; children must be made aware of the reduction of the time devote in front of an electronic entertainment device; encourage young people to devote more time to physical activity outside of school. It is the responsibility of local elected officials and non-profit associations to devote a few hours during the week to girls, adolescents and adult women in stadiums, sports halls and municipal swimming pools, to initiate a strategy to counteract overweight and obesity among women.

Our study is arguably limited by several aspects of design and analysis. Based on our small sample size, our findings may not generalize to all obese or overweight children in this country. Interest, the strength lies in the results which open the way to larger studies on children who live in large cities, or those who are confined during the long months of COVID-19.

Acknowledgements

The authors would like to thank the anonymous reviewers and the editor for their insightful comments and suggestions.

Conflict of interest

The authors declare that the research was conducted in the absence of any commercial or financial relationships that could be construed as a potential conflict of interest.

Author contributions

NA and LH authors contributed equally to the ideas presented. SKMB and AL wrote the draft of the paper. All authors contributed to editing the final version and approved the submitted version.

Author details

Nasreddine Aissaoui[1*], Lamia Hamaizia[1], Said Khalfa Mokhtar Brika[2], and Ahmed Laamari[3]

1 Faculty of Economics, Department of Finance Sciences, Business and Management Sciences, Oum El Bouaghi University, Algeria

2 Departement of Administrative Sciences, AppliedCollege, University of Bisha, Bisha, Saudi Arabia

3 Faculty of Science and Art in Al-Namas, University of Bisha, Bisha, Saudi Arabia

*Address all correspondence to: aissaoui.nasreddine@univ-oeb.dz

References

[1] WHO. Obésité et surpoids. World Health Organization 2020. [Internet]. 2020. Available from: https://www.who.int/fr/news-room/fact-sheets/detail/obesity-and-overweight. [Accessed: March 5, 2022]

[2] Thibault H, Rolland-Cachera MF. Stratégies de prévention de l'obésité chez l'enfant [Prevention strategies of childhood obesity]. Archives de pediatrie: organe officiel de la Societe francaise de pediatrie. 2003;**10**(12):1100-1108. DOI: 10.1016/j.arcped.2003.07.008

[3] Sahoo K, Sahoo B, Choudhury AK, Sofi NY, Kumar R, Bhadoria AS. Childhood obesity: Causes and consequences. Journal of Family Medicine and Primary Care. 2015;**4**(2):187-192. DOI: 10.4103/2249-4863.154628

[4] Di Cesare M, Sorić M, Bovet P, et al. The epidemiological burden of obesity in childhood: A worldwide epidemic requiring urgent action. BMC Medicine. 2019;**17**:212. DOI: 10.1186/s12916-019-1449-8

[5] Musung JM, Muyumba EK, Nkulu DN, Kakoma PK, Mukuku O, Kamalo BKM, et al. Prévalence du surpoids et de l'obésité chez l'adolescent en milieu scolaire à Lubumbashi, République Démocratique du Congo [prevalence of overweight and obesity among adolescents in school in Lubumbashi, Democratic Republic of Congo]. The Pan African Medical Journal. 2019;**32**:49. DOI: 10.11604/pamj.2019.32.49.15969

[6] INSP. Obésité en Algérie: 50% des hommes et un tiers des femmes souffrent de surpoids. Statistiques de l'Institut national de santé publique. [Internet]. 2021. Available from: https://radioalgerie.dz/news/fr/article/20210305/208110.html. [Accessed: March 7, 2022]

[7] Kumar S, Kelly AS. Review of childhood obesity: From epidemiology, etiology, and comorbidities to clinical assessment and treatment. Mayo Clinic Proceedings. 2017;**92**(2):251-265. DOI: 10.1016/j.mayocp.2016.09.017

[8] Cole TJ, Bellizi MC, Flegal KM, Dietz WH. Establishing a standard definition for child overweight and obesity worldwide: International survey. BMJ (Clinical Research ed.). 2000;**320**(7244):1240-1243. DOI: 10.1136/bmj.320.7244.1240

[9] Rolland-Cachera MF, Cole TJ, Sempé M, Tichet J, Rossignol C, Charraud A. Body mass index variations: Centiles from birth to 87 years. European Journal of Clinical Nutrition. 1991 Jan;**45**(1):13-21

[10] Arslan HN, Dundar C, Terzi Ö. Prevalence of overweight and obesity among school children and parents: A cross-sectional study. Rural and Remote Health. 2021;**21**(4):6773. DOI: 10.22605/RRH6773

[11] Taleb S, Agli AN. Obésité de l'enfant: rôle des facteurs socioéconomiques, obésité parentale, comportement alimentaire et activité physique, chez des enfants scolarisés dans une ville de l'Est algérien. Cahiers de Nutrition et de Diététique. 2009;**44**:198-206. DOI: 10.1016/j.cnd.2009.04.003

[12] Raiah M, Talhi R, Mesli MF. Surpoids et obésité des enfants de six à onze ans : prévalence et facteurs associés à Oran. Santé Publique. 2012;**24**:561-571. DOI: 10.3917/spub.126.0561

[13] Aspray TJ, Mugusi F, Rashid S, Whiting D, Edwards R, Alberti KG, et al. Essential non-communicable

disease health intervention project. Rural and urban differences in diabetes prevalence in Tanzania: The role of obesity, physical inactivity and urban living. Transactions of the Royal Society of Tropical Medicine and Hygiene. 2000;**94**(6):637-644. DOI: 10.1016/s0035-9203(00)90216-5

[14] Daepp MI, Gortmaker SL, Wang YC, Long MW, Kenney EL. WIC food package changes: Trends in childhood obesity prevalence. Pediatrics. 2019;**143**(5):e20182841. DOI: 10.1542/peds.2018-2841

[15] Regaieg S, Charfi N, Trabelsi L, Kamoun M, Feki H, Yaich S, et al. Prevalence and risk factors of overweight and obesity in a population of school children in urban areas Sfax, Tunisia. The Pan African Medical Journal. 2014;**17**:57. DOI: 10.11604/pamj.2014.17.57.3351

[16] Bhave S, Bavdekar A, Otiv M. IAP National Task Force for childhood prevention of adult diseases: Childhood obesity. IAP National Task Force for childhood prevention of adult diseases: Childhood obesity. IndianPediatr. 2004;**41**(6):559-575

[17] Corica D, Aversa T, Valenzise M, Messina MF, Alibrandi A, De Luca F, et al. Does family history of obesity, cardiovascular, and metabolic diseases influence onset and severity of childhood obesity? Frontiers in Endocrinology. 2018;**9**:187. DOI: 10.3389/fendo.2018.00187

[18] Saker M, Merzouk H, Merzouk SA, Ahmed SB, Narce M. Predictive factors of obesity and their relationships to dietary intake in schoolchildren in Western Algeria. Maedica (Bucur). 2011;**6**(2):90-99

[19] INSERM. Obésité ; dépistage et prévention chez l'enfant. Institut National de la Santé et de la Recherche Médicale 2000. Paris: Les éditions Inserm; 2000. p. XVIII-325. (Expertise collective). [Internet]. Available from: http://hdl.handle.net/10608/187. [Accessed: March 1, 2022]

[20] Kansra AR, Lakkunarajah S, Jay MS. Childhood and adolescent obesity: A review. Frontiers in Pediatrics. 2021;**8**:581461. DOI: 10.3389/fped.2020.581461

[21] Zitsman JL, Digiorgi MF, Kopchinski JS, Sysko R, Lynch L, Devlin M, et al. Adolescent gastric banding: A 5-year longitudinal study. Obesity Surgery. 2020;**30**(3):828-836. DOI: 10.1007/s11695-019-04321-5

[22] Galmés S, Serra F, Palou A. Vitamin E metabolic effects and genetic variants: A challenge for precision nutrition in obesity and associated disturbances. Nutrients. 2018;**10**(12):1919. DOI: 10.3390/nu10121919

Section 2

Clinical Aspects of Eating Disorders

Chapter 4

Clinical Aspects of Anorexia and Bulimia in Men

Val Bellman

Abstract

Men account for approximately 20% of people with Anorexia Nervosa (AN) and 30% of people with Bulimia Nervosa (BN). The clinical features of eating disorders (EDs) in men and women have many similarities but also some interesting and important differences. Men with eating disorders face persistent stigmatization because of the stereotype that EDs are "female" conditions. Most structured risk assessment tools for AN/BN likely reinforce gender stereotypes by better reflecting female symptoms. Moreover, gender similarities and differences in EDs have received scant investigation. Clearly, this form of disordered eating can put men in danger of experiencing a wide range of negative outcomes. Due to this lack of knowledge, these patients usually go undiagnosed and undertreated for ten or more years. These clinical differences are evident in the processes related to treatment initiation, retention, completion, and outcomes. Therefore, we discussed how the manifestation and progression of male eating disorders can be influenced by social context, including family and work relationships, interactions with social institutions. Treatment recommendations are discussed in the context of gender-based physiological differences, behavioral differences, comorbidities, and men-specific conditions.

Keywords: anorexia, bulimia, men, gender-specific aspects, rehabilitation

1. Introduction

Eating disorders (EDs) are complicated conditions that are multifactorial and affect individuals of any age or gender [1]. Historically, the stereotype of individuals with EDs has been affluent, middle-class, Caucasian female adolescents; however, the incidence of EDs in males is increasing, yet there is a disproportionate representation of males in ED research and clinical guidelines [2]. These illnesses are associated with personal, familial, and societal costs, with Anorexia Nervosa (AN) and Bulimia Nervosa (BN) being classified as two common EDs in the male population [3].

2. Epidemiology

Roughly 10 million males in the United States will experience an ED throughout their lifetime. In a study that included 36,000 adults in the U.S., the ED lifetime incidence in men was approximately 1.2%. In Canada, males account for up to 20% of ED cases, while males account for 20–25% of ED cases in the UK. These numbers may be even greater, as men may experience feelings of shame surrounding their ED because of the stigma associated with the condition. Traditionally, EDs are thought only to be present in females. Therefore, having an ED as a male may feel emasculating, preventing many men from seeking treatment and support for their illness [1].

The frequency of these different EDs in males varies across studies. For example, the literature demonstrates that females are three times likelier to have BED, while other research indicates that males make up to 40 percent of all BED cases. Regardless, BED is much more prevalent in males than AN or BN. Additionally, male EDs sometimes present with what is known as muscle dysmorphia, which refers to the societal ideal that men should be highly muscular with low body fat. Men seeking this appearance may engage in strict disordered eating, which can eventually lead to an ED [1].

AN is typically associated with having an emaciated and thin figure, specifically in females. Men, however, usually prefer a more muscular and lean appearance over appearing thin. Likewise, only 4.9 percent of high school boys overvalue body weight compared to 24.3 percent of girls of the same age. However, AN can still occur in men, and AN screening and definitions do not always consider how AN presentation may differ in men [3].

For example, the Diagnostic and Statistical Manual of Mental Disorders (DSM) historically excluded males from an AN diagnosis, and until 2013, amenorrhea was a diagnostic criterion [2]. Endocrine dysfunction is another female-specific criterion that has since been removed [3]. On the other hand, BN has a lifetime prevalence of up to 1.6 percent in males. Among all BN cases, males account for roughly one-third of all cases [3]. BN most commonly presents in males as excessive exercise, as opposed to laxative use or vomiting, which is more frequently seen in females [2].

3. Clinical presentations

Research has demonstrated that the symptoms of EDs among males are as severe as females; hence, it is important for clinicians to implement more screening and education efforts among males who have EDs. In a study assessing the 5.5-year outcome of AN in male versus female adolescent inpatients, it was found that both genders follow a similar course: Both have a similar age at admission, age at ED onset, and duration of illness [4]. Another study showed that the onset of AN in men occurs between the ages of 14–18 years, while bulimia occurs at the late stage of adulthood. Unfortunately, most screening strategies focus on thinness-oriented behaviors and caloric restriction and do not consider male-specific eating patterns and differences in body image and self-perception. Men's average scores on the ED screening scales are always lower than women's—even though they receive the same standardized tests and adequate attention during the evaluation process [5, 6].

The Diagnostic and Statistical Manual of Mental Disorders, fifth edition (DSM-5) contains diagnostic criteria for mental health disorders [1]. The criteria for AN and BN are summarized in **Table 1**.

The DSM-5 also includes severity specifiers (i.e., mild, moderate, severe, extreme) for AN and BN, which are determined by weight status (AN) and frequency of inappropriate compensatory behaviors (BN) [1]. **Table 2** summarizes the severity specifiers for both EDs.

The revisions in the DSM 5 addressed the clinical utility of a diagnostic criteria set for EDs, allowing more male patients to be properly diagnosed [7, 8].

	Anorexia Nervosa	Bulimia Nervosa
1.	Restriction of energy intake relative to requirements leading to a significantly low body weight in the context of age, sex, developmental trajectory, and physical health.	• Recurrent episodes of binge eating: • Eating in a discrete period (e.g., within any two-hour period), an amount of food that is definitely larger than most people eat during a similar period and under similar circumstances. • A sense of lack of control overeating during the episode (e.g., a feeling that one cannot stop eating or control what or how much one is eating).
2.	Intense fear of gaining weight or becoming fat, even though underweight.	Recurrent inappropriate compensatory behavior to prevent weight gain, such as self-induced vomiting, misuse of laxatives, diuretics, or other medications, fasting, or excessive exercise.
3.	Disturbance in the way in which one's body weight or shape is experienced, undue influence of body weight or shape on selfevaluation, or denial of the seriousness of the current low body weight.	The binge eating and inappropriate compensatory behaviors both occur, on average, at least once a week for 3 months.
4.	Two subtypes: 1. Restricting type 2. Binge eating/purging type	Self-evaluation is unduly influenced by body shape and weight.
5.	Even if all the DSM-5 TR criteria for anorexia are not met, a serious eating disorder can still be present. Atypical anorexia includes individuals who meet the criteria for anorexia but who are not underweight, despite significant weight loss. Individuals with atypical AN may experience many physiological complications associated with AN.	The disturbance does not occur exclusively during episodes of AN.

Table 1.
Diagnostic criteria for AN and BN.

Level of severity	Anorexia Nervosa (BMI)	Bulimia Nervosa
Mild	>17 kg/m^2	An average of 1–3 episodes of inappropriate compensatory behaviors per week
Moderate	16–16.99 kg/m^2	An average of 4–7 episodes of inappropriate compensatory behaviors per week
Severe	15–15.99 kg/m^2	An average of 8–13 episodes of inappropriate compensatory behaviors per week
Extreme	<15 kg/m^2	An average of 14 or more episodes of inappropriate compensatory behaviors per week

Table 2.
Severity specifiers for AN and BN.

Anorexia Nervosa in men	Bulimia Nervosa in men
Dietary restrictions among males with AN are usually focused on leanness with a goal to improve muscle definition and body shape [11]	Lots of similar patterns with regards to medical complications but later age of onset (18–26 years) [18]
The pathological preoccupation with weightlifting and strict adherence to eating foods that lower weight, not feeling muscular enough ("bigorexia") [12]	Premorbid obesity [21]
Men are more concerned about shape while female patients tend to be more focused on their weight [13]	Men prefer high protein and high fat content foods during binge-eating episodes [22]
Compulsive exercises and/or anxiety associated with missing a workout is often the last symptom to resolve, and the first sign of relapse [6]	Male patients tend to report eating large amounts of food and/or eating more often. Experiencing loss of control, distress, or somatic complaints due to binge eating tend to be underreported [23, 24]
Decreased interest in sex and low testosterone levels with associated behavioral changes [14]	Men tend to engage in non-purging compensatory behaviors [6]
The binge-purging subtype of AN is more common in men [15]	Overeating or binging on a cheat day or meal followed by a period of rigid dietary restriction [25]
Men may have a higher BMI among patients with AN [15]	Spitting of food as compensatory behavior in men with BN [26, 27]
Hospitalized boys with AN tend to be medically compromised (e.g., extremely low BMI and large orthostatic shifts in heart rate and blood pressure) [16]	Less concerned about their binge-eating behaviors and less preoccupied with weight control measures [28]
Adult males who are hospitalized for AN exhibit even more severe medical complications, with very high levels of osteopenia and osteoporosis [17]	Higher rates of psychiatric comorbidities (e.g., depression and anxiety) and substance use [18]
Frequently present like females but with higher rates of comorbid substance use and psychiatric disorders [18]	Possibly increased prevalence of homosexual or bisexual orientation [29, 30]
The duration of hospitalization for AN in males was shorter, and male patients had fewer suicide attempts (vs. female patients) [19]	Men who struggle with binge-eating disorder may develop bulimia if purging is used to cope with the fear of weight gain
Cortical atrophy on CT [20]	Central role of the frontostriatal area as its decreased activation in BN contributes to the severity of illness [31]

Table 3.
Characteristics of AN and BN in men.

Males are often unaware that their eating patterns and associated behaviors are characteristic of an ED [9]. They tend to develop a pattern of binging and purging behaviors, commonly described as coping mechanisms with daily stressors [10].

Many men report that they put off going to their PCP for as long as possible, even when they are experiencing life-threatening symptoms. They also tend to ignore mental health problems and seek help less often than women for mental health challenges [2]. The gender-specific characteristics of AN vs. BN are summarized in **Table 3**.

Both genders, male and female, with EDs were found to have a similar level of unhappiness with themselves. As EDs involve a major focus on weight, body shape, fat percentage, and distribution, they lead to dangerous behavioral adaptations. A lack of gender-appropriate information and resources for men with EDs as an additional stressor has been reported in the literature [32].

In another study that reported on the mortality of DSM-IV EDs among a large sample of males aged 16–61 and females aged 14–65, mortality rates for males were higher than in females, respectively, for AN and BN [33]. It was also found that compared to females, males with anorexia or bulimia showed shorter survival times. In the AN study, remission after 5.5 years was more frequent in males than in females [4]. Also, males with AN were found to have a shorter duration of ED and a shorter period of inpatient treatment [4].

4. Medical and psychiatric comorbidities in men with EDs

Men with ED suffer from many psychiatric disorders (including anxiety, depression, post-traumatic stress disorder (PTSD), and substance abuse) compared to the general population. Male EDs and related comorbidities are often underdiagnosed, undertreated, and misunderstood by many clinicians [34]. Moreover, men with AN and psychiatric comorbidity may exhibit a ninefold increase in mortality if left untreated [35].

Previous studies of men with ED have found that 56–95% of patients with an ED also receive a diagnosis for at least one more psychiatric disorder. The prevalence of psychiatric comorbidity in men with ED ranges widely from 2 to 27% for depression [36, 37] and 32–43% for anxiety disorders [37, 38]. Research has also demonstrated that up to 36% of male veterans with AN are diagnosed with schizophrenia or other psychotic disorders [39]. Other psychiatric comorbidities associated with AN include PTSD, substance use disorders, sexual dysfunction, and self-harming behaviors.

The most common psychiatric comorbidities of BN include MDD (50%), phobias (50%), PTSD (45%), attention-deficit/hyperactivity disorder (ADHD) (35%) [40], personality disorders (31%), anxiety disorders, and substance use problems (overall 61%, including 46% alcohol and 20% cocaine) [29]. Other authors have also reported similar rates of psychiatric comorbidity for men versus women with BN [36, 39].

Studies have shown that about 30% of male patients who have had EDs have been sexually abused in the past. These childhood traumatic experiences cause overall dissatisfaction with appearance and distort eating behaviors in the male population [41, 42]. Finally, 17% of patients with BN reported having suicidal thoughts, so identifying other commodities with EDs is necessary for the treatment of the disease [43].

While EDs can result in significant medical complications within every body system, the greatest impact on health is often observed in the cardiovascular, neurological, and skeletal systems. **Table 4** summarizes the comorbid somatic conditions and syndromes associated with AN and BN in men.

Category of symptoms and/or syndromes	Description
General somatic changes	Clinically significant fluctuations in weight and BMI Weakness, fatigue, lethargy Heat/cold intolerance Diaphoresis and/or hyperhidrosis Dizziness, vertigo, syncope/presyncope
Oropharyngeal symptoms	Oral trauma, cuts, lacerations Dental erosion and caries Salivary gland enlargement
Cardiopulmonary symptoms	Chest pain, palpitations, chest discomfort Arrhythmias, bradycardia, prolonged QTc Orthostatic BP changes, hypotension, and tachycardia Shortness of breath Edema (localized vs. generalized)
Gastrointestinal symptoms	GI discomfort/distress Bloating, meteorism Early satiety (fullness) Reflux with/without heartburn Hematemesis Hemorrhoids and rectal prolapse Constipation or diarrhea
Endocrinopathies and hormonal changes	Hypoglycemia Hypogonadism and infertility Stress fractures Osteopenia
Neurological symptoms	Confusion, disorientation Amnesia Cognitive deficits Seizures
Dermatological symptoms	Lanugo, alopecia Carotenoderma Russell sign Poor wound healing Brittle hair/nails

Table 4.
Somatic signs and symptoms of AN and BN in male patients.

5. Special considerations

5.1 Sports and eating disorders

In sports, low body weight and leanness are often regarded as advantageous from a performance perspective. This can be observed in endurance-based sports (e.g., distance running and cycling), weight-based sports (e.g., wrestling and jockeys), anti-gravitational sports (e.g., long jump and high jump), and others where leanness has been associated with improved performance outcomes [44]. Sometimes, sport-related requirements place an unnecessary burden on athletes, resulting in the increased likelihood of developing EDs [45–47].

EDs are especially common in bodybuilding, as it promotes leanness and muscularity as a method of scoring and performance and encourages the development of exercise and nutrition-related behaviors that may adversely affect one's overall mental health.

A recent scoping review examined the prevalence of male athletes reporting disordered symptoms, subclinical EDs, and clinical EDs; prevalence rates ranged from 0 to 85.5%, 1.5–11.0%, and 1.3–32.5%, respectively [48]. Furthermore, the prevalence of EDs in male weight-sensitive sports versus less weight-sensitive sports ranged from 5 to 50% and 0–31%, respectively [49–53]. Interestingly, the prevalence of EDs among the general male population was only 2.2% (range, 0.8–6.5i%) [54].

Men who exhibit behaviors associated with a negative body image (e.g., body image dissatisfaction, preoccupation/obsession with specific body areas, body checking, and negative self-talk), or have psychological or personality features such as low self-esteem, fear of negative evaluation, depression, and impulsivity may be at an increased risk of EDs [44, 55–58]. Further, socio-cultural factors, such as the ideal male body size/shape (i.e, muscular, lean, and V-shaped physique [broad shoulders and narrow waist]), also contribute to the increased propensity for EDs. This is further pronounced in male sports, whereas outward and physical appearances can impact perceptions related to performance [44, 48].

5.2 Role of sexual orientation

When looking at the possibly distinct viewpoints of males with EDs, one thing to explore is their self-perceived sexual orientation. According to research, LGBTQ adults and youths are more prone to developing mental illnesses because of the increased stress generated by prejudice and stigma [59].

Most characteristics of males and females with EDs appear to be similar; however, homosexuality or bisexuality appears to be a risk factor in males, specifically for those with BN. In a study conducted at Massachusetts General Hospital, 42% of male bulimic patients were identified as either homosexual or bisexual, and 58% of anorexic patients were identified as asexual [28]. Biologically, there may be similarities in brain structure between homosexual men and heterosexual women, and homosexual men may react to environmental stressors in a feminine way, thus increasing their risk of EDs [28].

Because of stigma, prejudice, and proximal stresses, homosexuality plays a role in males' appearance and the progression, or severity of EDs. As a result, they have been largely ignored in therapy and diagnosis, contributing to the disorder's severity [34]. ED stereotypes impede the provision of evidence-based treatment for males, thus falling short of the success of gender-specific conditions. Compared to females with EDs, the general population may see men with ED as gay or bisexual and label them as "weak" or mentally disabled. Males are expected to hide their weaknesses in today's environment, especially shame and despair, which relate to the stigma of being "feminine." In homosexual and bisexual males, "minority" stress and stigma are also linked to binge eating behaviors [59].

Reportedly, 54% of LGBT male teenagers have been diagnosed with EDs [60]. They are caught in a vicious loop of exercising for weight reduction to improve their health, only to end up on a "runaway diet" that leads to self-starvation [60].

5.3 Identification, assessment, and differential diagnosis

Risks of disordered eating and associated clinical EDs should not be discounted among male patients, and increased vigilance regarding the screening and subsequent management of both subclinical and clinical conditions is warranted. Male EDs are present in a range of settings, and collateral information should be obtained to justify

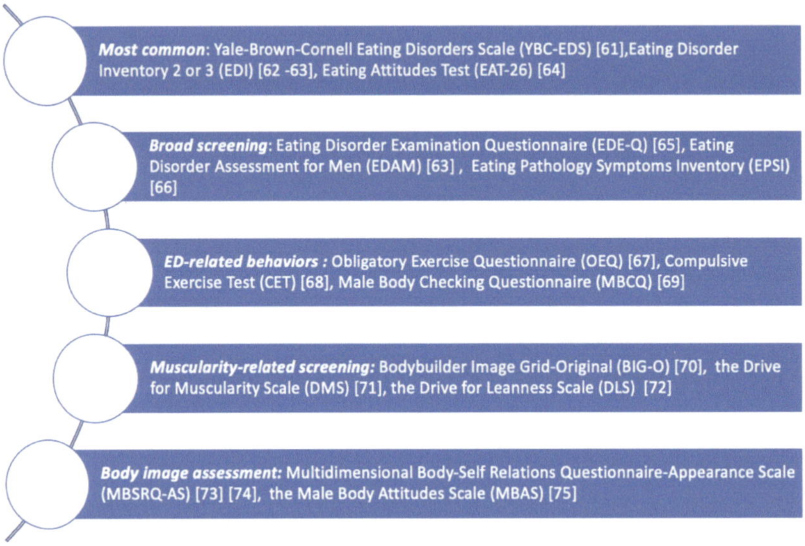

Figure 1.
Standardized rating scales for EDs in men [61–75].

the diagnosis. Underreporting ED symptoms impedes appropriate diagnosis, treatment, and research in this area.

When assessing an eating disorder, the clinician is expected to use all available methods to determine whether a male patient has an eating disorder. However, standardized diagnostic tools should not be used as the main screening method due to challenges with reliability and variability in clinical presentations. **Figure 1** outlines the standardized rating scales for EDs in men.

It is recommended to avoid using single measures such as BMI, the degree of weight loss/gain or duration of illness in the justification of the diagnosis. General medical conditions and other psychiatric disorders can simulate the binging, purging behaviors, disturbed food intake, and other compensatory reactions seen in EDs. Healthcare providers are expected to assess patients' physical health, the possibility of underdiagnosed medical conditions, and evaluate the risk factors associated with disturbed eating behaviors.

Figure 2 outlines the differential diagnoses of AN and BN in accordance with their presentations.

Approaching EDs using a multidisciplinary approach (e.g., the inclusion of a healthcare provider, dietitian, mental health specialist, etc.) allows for a patient-centered approach to care and should be prioritized. Sometimes, men with AN and BN may require a higher level of care due to medical instability. These challenging patients require a unique collaboration between many specialists, and general hospital units or inpatient psychiatric facilities may not be set up to provide appropriate care. The decision to hospitalize should be made only when all psychiatric and medical factors are considered. One of the most important factors is a progressive decline in oral intake and weight despite interventions, a history of weight instability, and comorbid psychiatric and/or medical conditions.

More than 50% of male adolescents with EDs who present to the clinic for treatment result in the need for immediate hospitalization due to significant delays in treatment [76]. The American Academy of Pediatrics released the criteria for

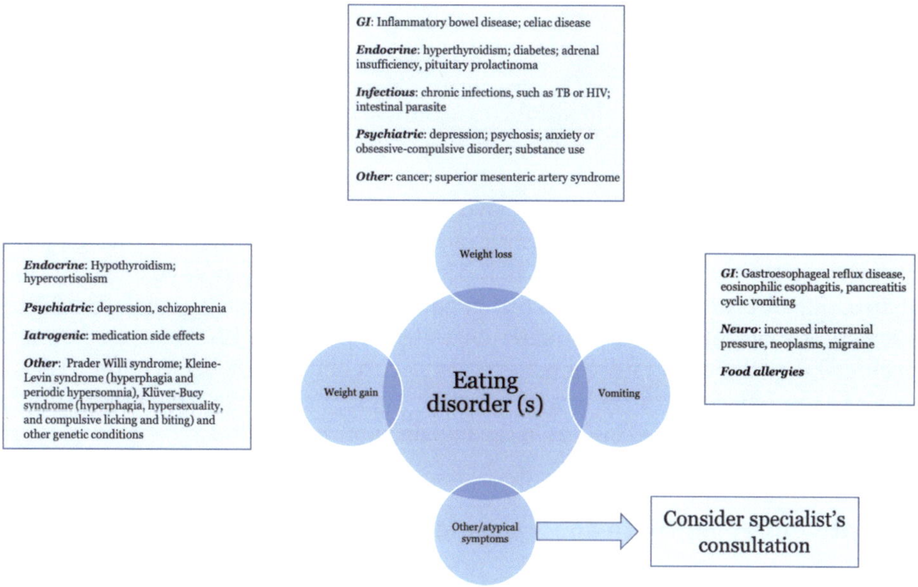

Figure 2.
Differential diagnosis of AN and BN in men.

inpatient treatment in 2014 [77]. Unfortunately, gender-specific criteria for hospitalization are still unavailable. Generally speaking, the patient is expected to be hospitalized when one or more of the following criteria are met:

1. <75% median BMI for age and sex

2. Dehydration

3. Electrolyte disturbances (hypokalemia, hyponatremia, or hypophosphatemia)

4. ECG abnormalities (e.g., prolonged QTc or severe bradycardia)

5. Physiologic instability

    a. Severe bradycardia (HR <50 BPM daytime; <45 BPM at night)

    b. Hypotension (90/45 mm Hg)

    c. Hypothermia (body temperature, 96°F, 35.6°C)

    d. Orthostatic hypotension

6. Failure of outpatient treatment

7. Acute or persistent food refusal

8. Uncontrollable binge eating and purging

9. Acute medical complications of malnutrition (e.g., syncope, seizures, cardiac failure, pancreatitis, etc.)

10. Unstable psychiatric or medical comorbidity that cannot be treated on an outpatient basis

As many as half of patients who survive hospitalization for ED experience prolonged work absence, financial difficulty, or emotional effects, each of which may further impede recovery. Iwajomo et al. reported that mortality after hospitalization for an eating disorder was five times higher compared to the general population [78]. Specifically, mortality rates were higher for males with AN and BN. Other authors also concluded that mortality rates for male patients with BN were higher than for their female counterparts [79]. Finally, a recent study confirmed that inpatient mortality for males with AN was twice as high as in the female population [80].

6. Treatment of men with anorexia and bulimia

The goal of the treatment is to attain improved eating habits and overall physical and psychological well-being. In the treatment process for an ED, one of the first steps is understanding and admitting that the patient has an ED and identifying the need for a change. EDs in men may remain unidentified and undiagnosed as men are prone to hiding their symptoms due to the fear of judgment and shame of having a female disease [34]. It is important to raise public awareness about male EDs and to help motivate male patients to accept and get help.

Studies show a significant difference between the health of men and the health of women, as men are less likely to seek treatment for mental health problems. Many male patients with AN or BN tend to underuse professional services, despite their susceptibility to these types of illnesses. Most male patients deny that they are sick, resist treatment (usually medication and/or talk therapy), and demonstrate indirect support-seeking patterns (e.g., pushed into treatment by spouse) [81].

Multidisciplinary care teams consisting of a physician, dietician, and mental health providers are encouraged. Healthcare providers play a key role in the detection of EDs in men, as they are the first professionals men encounter. Stabilizing nutrition and weight in the early phases of recovery and searching for balance between rest, sleep, and activity are also crucial steps [81]. Interpersonal changes, especially in acquiring more flexibility in social relations, and learning how to distance from difficult relationships, may also be helpful. Another important step is being able to better recognize and understand one's own personal needs, and have increased self-care and self-regulation, as that can help with opening up strict cognitive schemas, and ultimately lead to a better relationship with food [81].

Unfortunately, there are no gender-specific practice guidelines or standards of care for men with EDs [6]. **Table 5** summarizes the general treatment guidelines for anorexia and bulimia.

The traditional treatment for ED has largely been female-focused and sometimes unsuited for men, as they require a gender-sensitized treatment approach [32].

Level of Intervention	American Psychiatric Association (APA) [82]	World Federation of Societies of Biological Psychiatry (WFSBP) [83]	The National Institute for Health and Care Excellence's (NICE) [84]
Anorexia Nervosa			
First-line	• Nutritional rehabilitation: restore weight, adjust eating pattern with a goal to achieve consistent weight gain 2–3 lb./week for hospitalized patients and 0.5–1 lb. in outpatient setting • Psychosocial interventions • Promotility agents (e.g., metoclopramide) for bloating and abdominal discomfort that occur during refeeding	No clear evidence to combine psychotherapy with pharmacotherapy	• Psychoeducation with eating disorder focused CBT, Maudsley Anorexia Nervosa for adults, or specialist supportive clinical malnutrition • For children and young people, psychotherapy with AN-focused family therapy • No hyperfocus on medications • Consider the impact of malnutrition on medications
Second-line	• SSRI are not advantageous for weight gain in patients who are receiving inpatient treatment • SSRI in combination with psychotherapy are recommended for persistent depressive, anxiety and/or obsessive- compulsive disorder (OCD)-like symptoms • Second generation antipsychotics may be considered in patients with treatment-resistant inability to gain weight, severe obsessional/delusional thinking and denial	• Adjunctive pharmacotherapy for comorbid conditions • Olanzapine may be considered for weight gain • Low-dose quetiapine may cause improvement with minimal side effects • Prokinetic agents may improve gastric emptying • Zinc supplements may improve weight gain and affective symptoms	• Adults: psychotherapy with eating disorder focused focal psychodynamic therapy • Children/young adults: ED-focused CBT; adolescent-focused psychotherapy for AN

Level of Intervention	American Psychiatric Association (APA) [82]	World Federation of Societies of Biological Psychiatry (WFSBP) [83]	The National Institute for Health and Care Excellence's (NICE) [84]
Bulimia Nervosa			
First-line	• Nutritional rehabilitation • Psychosocial interventions: CBT, interpersonal therapy, family therapy • SSRI are safe and effective: fluoxetine is FDA approved for BN. • Dosages of SSRIs are higher than those used for depression	• Fluoxetine is the best studies option for patients with BN • Antidepressants should be used in doses higher than those required for depression	• BN-focused guided self-help • Children/young adults: Individual psycho-therapy with BN-focused family therapy • Avoid overprescribing medications • Consider the impact of malnutrition and compensatory behaviors
Second-line	• IPT is recom-mended for patients who do not respond to CBT • SSRIs/SNRls might be helpful for comorbid condi-tions, obsessions, and some impulse disorder symptoms	• Fluvoxamine and sertraline are good alternatives • Topiramate decreases binge behavior with a moderate risk-to-benefit ratio • Ondansetron has efficacy over placebos	• Individual BN-focused psychotherapy • Children/young adults: psychotherapy with individual BN-focused CBT

Table 5.
Treatment guidelines for AN and BN.

However, some authors have concluded that male and female patients may benefit equally from the same types of therapy [34]. Nevertheless, men want to be treated with dignity and with an acknowledgment of their value as individuals. Many of them do not want to be treated differently because of gender. One of the most widely cited elements of disrespect mentioned by patients is simply failing to pay attention to their needs by leaving them unattended or ignored [85].

Some patients believe that receiving a formal diagnosis can boost their self-image and self-esteem and motivate them to continue treatment [86]. Moreover, good quality therapeutic alliance is one of the most robust predictors of positive treatment outcomes in men with EDs—which is typically a reduction of primary symptoms of EDs [32]. Male patients who are actively engaged in treatment demonstrate improvements in their symptoms and quality of life. Interestingly, success rates are generally higher for men than women [87, 88]. The stigma of men with EDs and body image issues has yet to be overcome.

Gender-specific treatment groups can be considered an important treatment option: sensitive to all of these issues and addressing the unique needs of each patient in a comfortable and supportive environment [85]. Interestingly, most male patients prefer mixed-gender treatment groups [85]. Although gender mismatching (male patient-female therapist) does not impair the therapeutic alliance, male psychotherapists can bring that male-to-male relationship into the treatment process, and that can be extremely transformative. Male patients may need to have therapeutic interventions repeated multiple times before they understand why they are engaged in compulsive exercises or eating in a specific way. Thankfully, male patients with EDs who are engaged in recovery believe that therapy is the best investment that they have ever made [81].

It is important to discuss men's thinking about wanting to be highly muscular and other potential symptoms of body dysmorphic disorders. Not only do men see themselves as healthy, but most look very healthy from an outward perspective [34]. Research has shown that men with AN and BN disorders experience multiple problems with sexual functioning in both the physiological (e.g., erectile dysfunction) and psychological (e.g., anxiety) dimensions of sexuality [86]. When men enter the treatment process, they do not always give providers the chance to understand the reasoning behind these clinical symptoms and their risks and to find a potential solution. While the presence of erectile dysfunction may signal potentially serious medical conditions, EDs are frequently overlooked.

Despite the widespread penetration of specialized testing in health care, there has been no empirical research to date investigating the impact of quality of evidence on the strength of treatment recommendations for patients with EDs. Previous clinical recommendations for treating men with EDs also emphasized the role of testosterone [89] and genetic vulnerability [90]. However, neither factor is accurate enough at this stage to make individual predictions about how a person's symptoms will respond to treatment over time.

7. Conclusion

Demographic survey statistics show that around 10 million men and boys in the United States suffer from EDs and distorted eating practices. AN and BN affect persons of many identities; discrepancies have been discovered in specific marginalized groups, such as gender and sexual minorities. These patients experience various forms of stress, including significant stigma and social victimization. Moreover, men from various sexual minorities are overrepresented in the ED literature because they tend to seek treatment more often than the general population.

Men are disproportionately affected by EDs due to shame, social norms, and prejudice, all of which contribute to the manifestation, prognosis, and severity of bulimia and anorexia. Moreover, underreporting ED symptoms impedes appropriate diagnosis, treatment, and research in this area.

Author details

Val Bellman[1,2]

1 Department of Psychiatry, University of Missouri Kansas City, Kansas City, MO, USA

2 California Southern University, Costa Mesa, CA, USA

*Address all correspondence to: val.bellmanmd@gmail.com

References

[1] American Psychiatric Association. Diagnostic and Statistical Manual of Mental Disorders. 5th ed. Washington, DC: American Psychiatric Association; 2013

[2] Sangha S, Oliffe JL, Kelly MT, McCuaig F. Eating Disorders in Males: How Primary Care Providers Can Improve Recognition, Diagnosis, and Treatment. American Journal of Men's Health. 2019;**13**(3):1557988319857424. DOI: 10.1177/1557988319857424. Available from: https://www.ncbi.nlm.nih.gov/pmc/articles/PMC6560809/

[3] Gorrell S, Murray SB. Eating disorders in males. Child and Adolescent Psychiatric Clinics of North America. 2019;**28**(4):641-651. DOI: 10.1016/j.chc.2019.05.012

[4] Quadflieg N, Naab S, Voderholzer U, Fichter MM. Long-term outcome in males with anorexia nervosa: A prospective, sex-matched study. The International Journal of Eating Disorders. 2022;**55**(3):393-398. DOI: 10.1002/eat.23672

[5] Darcy AM, Doyle AC, Lock J, et al. The eating disorders examination in adolescent males with anoreia nervosa: How does it compare to adolescent females? The International Journal of Eating Disorders. 2012;**45**:110-114

[6] Murray SB, Nagata JM, Griffiths S, et al. The enigma of male eating disorders: A critical review and synthesis. Clinical Psychology Review. 2017;**57**:1-11

[7] Smink FR, van Hoeken D, Oldehinkel AJ, Hoek HW. Prevalence and severity of DSM-5 eating disorders in a community cohort of adolescents. The International Journal of Eating Disorders. 2014;**47**(6):610-619. DOI: 10.1002/eat.22316

[8] Raevuori A, Keski-Rahkonen A, Hoek HW. A review of eating disorders in males. Current Opinion in Psychiatry. 2014;**27**(6):426-430. DOI: 10.1097/YCO.0000000000000113

[9] MacCaughelty C, Wagner R, Rufino K. Does being overweight or male increase a patient's risk of not being referred for an eating disorder consult. International Journal of Eating Disorders. 2016;**49**(10):963-966. DOI: 10.1002/eat.22556

[10] Burnette CB, Simpson CC, Mazzeo SE. Exploring gender differences in the link between weight suppression and eating pathology. Eating Behaviors. 2017;**27**:17-22. DOI: 10.1016/j.eatbeh.2017.10.001

[11] Pope HG, Phillips KA, Olivardia R. The Adonis Complex: The Secret Crisis of Male Body Obsession. New York: The Free Press; 2000

[12] Mosley PE. Bigorexia: Bodybuilding and muscle dysmorphia. European Eating Disorders Review. 2009;**17**(3):191-198. DOI: 10.1002/erv.897

[13] Voges MM, Giabbiconi CM, Schöne B, Waldorf M, Hartmann AS, Vocks S. Gender differences in body evaluation: Do men show more self-serving double standards than women? Frontiers in Psychology. 2019;**12**(10):544. DOI: 10.3389/fpsyg.2019.00544

[14] Skolnick A, Schulman RC, Galindo RJ, Mechanick JI. The endocrinopathies of male anorexia nervosa: Case series. AACE Clinical Case Report. 2016;**2**(4):e351-e357. DOI: 10.4158/EP15945.CR

[15] Valente S, Di Girolamo G, Forlani M, et al. Sex-specific issues

in eating disorders: A clinical and psychopathological investigation. Eating and Weight Disorders. 2017;**22**(4):707-715. DOI: 10.1007/s40519-017-0432-7

[16] Coelho JS, Kumar A, Kilvert M, Kunkel L, Lam PY. Male youth with eating disorders: Clinical and medical characteristics of a sample of inpatients. Eating Disorders. 2015;**23**(5):455-461. DOI: 10.1080/10640266.2015.1027119

[17] Sabel AL, Rosen E, Mehler PS. Severe anorexia nervosa in males: Clinical presentations and medical treatment. Eating Disorders. 2014;**22**:209-220

[18] Muise AM, Stein DG, Arbess G. Eating disorders in adolescent boys: A review of the adolescent and young adult literature. The Journal of Adolescent Health. 2003;**33**(6):427-435. DOI: 10.1016/s1054-139x(03)00060-0

[19] Gueguen J, Godart N, Chambry J, et al. Severe anorexia nervosa in men: Comparison with severe AN in women and analysis of mortality. The International Journal of Eating Disorders. 2012;**45**(4):537-545. DOI: 10.1002/eat.20987

[20] Shapiro M, Davis AA, Nguyen ML. Severe anorexia nervosa in a 20-year-old male with pericardial effusion and cortical atrophy. International Journal of Psychiatry in Medicine. 2014;**48**(2):95-102. DOI: 10.2190/PM.48.2.b

[21] Shaw JA, Herzog DB, Clark VL, et al. Elevated pre-morbid weights in bulimic individuals are usually surpassed post-morbidly: Implications for perpetuation of the disorder. The International Journal of Eating Disorders. 2012;**45**(4):512-523. DOI: 10.1002/eat.20985

[22] Wansink B, Cheney MM, Chan N. Exploring comfort food preferences across age and gender. Physiology & Behavior. 2003;**79**(4-5):739-747. DOI: 10.1016/s0031-9384(03)00203-8

[23] Lewinsohn PM, Seeley JR, Moerk KC, Striegel-Moore RH. Gender differences in eating disorder symptoms in young adults. The International Journal of Eating Disorders. 2002;**32**(4):426-440. DOI: 10.1002/eat.10103

[24] Striegel-Moore RH, Rossello F, Perrin N, DeBar L, Wilson GT, May A, et al. Gender differences in the prevalence of eating disorder symptoms. International Journal of Eating Disorders. 2009;**42**(5):471-474

[25] Murray SB, Pila E, Mond JM, et al. Cheat meals: A benign or ominous variant of binge eating behavior? Appetite. 2018;**130**:274-278. DOI: 10.1016/j.appet.2018.08.026

[26] Guarda AS, Coughlin JW, Cummings M, et al. Chewing and spitting in eating disorders and its relationship to binge eating. Eating Behaviors. 2004;**5**(3):231-239. DOI: 10.1016/j.eatbeh.2004.01.001

[27] Fairburn CG, Cooper PJ. The clinical features of bulimia nervosa. The British Journal of Psychiatry. 1984;**144**:23-46. DOI: 10.1192/bjp.144.3.238

[28] Carlat DJ, Camargo CA Jr. Review of bulimia nervosa in males. The American Journal of Psychiatry. 1991;**148**(7):831-843. DOI: 10.1176/ajp.148.7.831

[29] Carlat DJ, Camargo CA Jr, Herzog DB. Eating disorders in males: A report on 135 patients. The American Journal of Psychiatry. 1997;**154**(8): 1127-1132. DOI: 10.1176/ajp.154.8.1127

[30] Bramon-Bosch E, Troop NA, Treasure JL. Eating disorders in males: A comparison with female patients. European Eating Disorders Review.

2000;**8**(4):321-328. DOI: 10.1002/1099-0968(200008)8:4<321:AID-ERV355>3.0.CO;2-G

[31] Skunde M et al. Neural signature of behavioral inhibition in women with bulimia nervosa. Journal of Psychiatry and Neuroscience. 2016;**41**(5):E69-E78. DOI: 10.1503/jpn.150335

[32] Räisänen U, Hunt K. The role of gendered constructions of eating disorders in delayed help-seeking in men: A qualitative interview study. BMJ Open. 2014;**4**:e004342. DOI: 10.1136/bmjopen-2013-004342

[33] Fichter MM, Naab S, Voderholzer U, Quadflieg N. Mortality in males as compared to females treated for an eating disorder: A large prospective controlled study. National Library of Medicine. 2021;**26**:1627-1637

[34] Strother E, Lemberg R, Stanford SC, Turberville D. Eating disorders in men: Underdiagnosed, undertreated, and misunderstood. Eating Disorders. 2012;**20**(5):346-355. DOI: 10.1080/10640266.2012.715512

[35] Kask J, Ramklint M, Kolia N, et al. Anorexia nervosa in males: Excess mortality and psychiatric co-morbidity in 609 Swedish in-patients. Psychological Medicine. 2017;**47**(8):1489-1499. DOI: 10.1017/S0033291717000034

[36] Woodside DB, Garfinkel PE, Lin E, Goering P, Kaplan AS, Goldbloom DS, et al. Comparisons of men with full or partial eating disorders, men without eating disorders, and women with eating disorders in the community. American Journal of Psychiatry. 2001;**158**:570-574

[37] Weltzin TE, Cornella-Carlson T, Fitzpatrick ME, Kennington B, Bean P, Jefferies C. Treatment issues and outcomes for males with eating disorders. Eating Disorders. 2012;**20**:444-459

[38] Feldman MB, Meyer IH. Comorbidity and age of onset of eating disorders in gay men, lesbians, and bisexuals. Psychiatry Research. 2010;**180**:126-131

[39] Striegel-Moore RH, Garvin V, Dohm FA, Rosenheck R. Psychiatric comorbidity of eating disorders in men: A national study of hospitalized veterans. International Journal of Eating Disorders. 2019;**25**(4):399-404. DOI: 10.1002/(SICI)1098-108X(199905)25:4<399::AID-EAT4>3.0.CO;2-0

[40] Hudson JI, Hiripi E, Pope HG Jr, Kessler RC. The prevalence and correlates of eating disorders in the National Comorbidity Survey Replication. Biological Psychiatry. 2007;**61**(3):348-358. DOI: 10.1016/j.biopsych.2006.03.040

[41] Connors ME, Morse W. Sexual abuse and eating disorders: A review. The International Journal of Eating Disorders. 1993;**13**(1):1-11. DOI: 10.1002/1098-108x(199301)13:1<1::aid-eat2260130102>3.0.co;2-p

[42] Morgan J. The Invisible Man: A Self-Help Guide for Men with Eating Disorders, Compulsive Exercise, and Bigorexia. New York, NY: Routledge; 2008

[43] Yao S, Kuja-Halkola R, Thornton LM, et al. Familial liability for eating disorders and suicide attempts: Evidence from a population registry in Sweden. JAMA Psychiatry. 2016;**73**(3):284-291. DOI: 10.1001/jamapsychiatry.2015.2737

[44] Eichstadt M, Luzier J, Cho D, Weisenmuller C. Eating disorders in male athletes. Sports Health. 2020;**12**(4):327-333. DOI: 10.1177/1941738120928991

[45] Griffiths S, Murray SB, Touyz S. Disordered eating and the muscular ideal. Journal of Eating Disorders. 2013;**1**:15. DOI: 10.1186/2050-2974-1-15

[46] Lavender JM, Brown TA, Murray SB. Men, muscles, and eating disorders: An overview of traditional and muscularity-oriented disordered eating. Current Psychiatry Reports. 2017;**19**(6):32. DOI: 10.1007/s11920-017-0787-5

[47] Ravaldi C, Vannacci A, Zucchi T, et al. Eating disorders and body image disturbances among ballet dancers, gymnasium users and body builders. Psychopathology. 2003;**36**(5):247-254. DOI: 10.1159/000073450

[48] Karrer Y, Halioua R, Mötteli S, et al. Disordered eating and eating disorders in male elite athletes: A scoping review. BMJ Open Sport & Exercise Medicine. 2020;**6**(1):e000801. DOI: 10.1136/bmjsem-2020-000801

[49] Currie A. Sport and eating disorders: Understanding and managing the risks. Asian Journal of Sports Medicine. 2010;**1**(2):63-68. DOI: 10.5812/asjsm.34864

[50] Sundgot-Borgen J, Torstveit MK. Prevalence of eating disorders in elite athletes is higher than in the general population. Clinical Journal of Sport Medicine. 2004;**14**(1):25-32. DOI: 10.1097/00042752-200401000-00005

[51] Byrne S, McLean N. Elite athletes: Effects of the pressure to be thin. Journal of Science and Medicine in Sport. 2002;**5**(2):80-94. DOI: 10.1016/s1440-2440(02)80029-9

[52] Rousselet M, Guérineau B, Paruit MC, et al. Disordered eating in French high-level athletes: Association with type of sport, doping behavior, and psychological features. Eating and Weight Disorder EWD. 2017;**22**(1):61-68. DOI: 10.1007/s40519-016-0342-0

[53] Rosendahl J, Bormann B, Aschenbrenner K, Aschenbrenner F, Strauss B. Dieting and disordered eating in German high school athletes and non-athletes. Scandinavian Journal of Medicine & Science in Sports. 2009;**19**(5):731-739. DOI: 10.1111/j.1600-0838.2008.00821.x

[54] Galmiche M, Déchelotte P, Lambert G, Tavolacci MP. Prevalence of eating disorders over the 2000-2018 period: A systematic literature review. The American Journal of Clinical Nutrition. 2019;**109**(5):1402-1413. DOI: 10.1093/ajcn/nqy342

[55] Goldfield GS, Blouin AG, Woodside DB. Body image, binge eating, and bulimia nervosa in male bodybuilders. Canadian Journal of Psychiatry Review and Canadian Psychiatry. 2006;**51**(3):160-168. DOI: 10.1177/070674370605100306

[56] Devrim A, Bilgic P, Hongu N. Is there any relationship between body image perception, eating disorders, and muscle dysmorphic disorders in male bodybuilders? American Journal of Men's Health. 2018;**12**(5):1746-1758. DOI: 10.1177/1557988318786868

[57] Stapleton P, McIntyre T, Bannatyne A. Body image avoidance, body dissatisfaction, and eating pathology: Is there a difference between male gym users and non-gym users? American Journal of Men's Health. 2016;**10**(2):100-109. DOI: 10.1177/1557988314556673

[58] Andersen RE, Barlett SJ, Morgan GD, Brownell KD. Weight loss, psychological, and nutritional patterns in competitive male body builders. The International

Journal of Eating Disorders. 1995;**18**(1):49-57. DOI: 10.1002/1098-108x(199507)18:1<49:aid-eat2260180106>3.0.co;2-c

[59] Parker LL, Harriger JA. A review of the literature reviews eating disorders and disordered eating behaviors in the LGBT population. Journal of Eating Disorders. 2020;**8**(1):51. DOI: 10.1186/s40337-020-00327-y

[60] Essayli JH, Murakami JM, Latner JD. Perceived sexual orientation of men and women with eating disorders and obesity. Journal of Homosexuality. 2018;**66**(6):735-745. DOI: 10.1080/00918369.2018.1484228

[61] Bellace DL, Tesser R, Berthod S, et al. The Yale-Brown-Cornell eating disorders scale self-report questionnaire: A new, efficient tool for clinicians and researchers. The International Journal of Eating Disorders. 2012;**45**(7):856-860. DOI: 10.1002/eat.22023

[62] Spillane NS, Boerner LM, Anderson KG, Smith GT. Comparability of the eating disorder Inventory-2 between women and men. Assessment. 2004;**11**(1):85-93. DOI: 10.1177/1073191103260623

[63] Stanford SC, Lemberg R. A clinical comparison of men and women on the eating disorder inventory-3 (EDI-3) and the eating disorder assessment for men (EDAM). Eating Disorders. 2012;**20**(5):379-394. DOI: 10.1080/10640266.2012.715516

[64] Papini NM, Jung M, Cook A, et al. Psychometric properties of the 26-item eating attitudes test (EAT-26): An application of rasch analysis. Journal of Eating Disorders. 2022;**10**:62. DOI: 10.1186/s40337-022-00580-3

[65] Fairburn CG, Beglin SJ. Assessment of eating disorders: Interview or self-report questionnaire? The International Journal of Eating Disorders. 1994;**16**(4):363-370

[66] Forbush KT, Wildes JE, Pollack LO, et al. Development and validation of the eating pathology symptoms inventory (EPSI). Psychological Assessment. 2013;**25**(3):859-878. DOI: 10.1037/a0032639

[67] Thompson KJ, Pasman L. The obligatory exercise questionnaire. Behavior Therapy. 1991;**14**:137

[68] Taranis L, Touyz S, Meyer C. Disordered eating and exercise: Development and preliminary validation of the compulsive exercise test (CET). European Eating Disorders Review. 2011;**19**(3):256-268. DOI: 10.1002/erv.1108

[69] Hildebrandt T, Walker DC, Alfano L, Delinsky S, Bannon K. Development and validation of a male-specific body checking questionnaire. The International Journal of Eating Disorders. 2010;**43**(1):77-87. DOI: 10.1002/eat.20669

[70] Hildebrandt T, Langenbucher J, Schlundt DG. Muscularity concerns among men: Development of attitudinal and perceptual measures. Body Image. 2004;**1**(2):169-181. DOI: 10.1016/j.bodyim.2004.01.001

[71] McCreary DR, Sasse DK. An exploration of the drive for muscularity in adolescent boys and girls. Journal of American College Health. 2000;**48**(6):297-304. DOI: 10.1080/07448480009596271

[72] Smolak L, Murnen SK. Drive for leanness: Assessment and relationship to gender, gender role and objectification. Body Image. 2008;**5**(3):251-260. DOI: 10.1016/j.bodyim.2008.03.004

[73] Brown TA, Cash TA, Mikulka PJ. Attitudinal body-image assessment: Factor analysis of the body-self relations questionnaire. Journal of Personality Assessment. 1990;**55**:135-144

[74] Pickett TC, Lewis RJ, Cash TF. Men, muscles, and body image: Comparisons of competitive bodybuilders, weight trainers, and athletically active controls. British Journal of Sports Medicine. 2005;**39**:217-222

[75] Tylka TL, Bergeron D, Schwartz JP. Development and psychometric evaluation of the male body attitudes scale (MBAS). Body Image. 2005;**2**(2):161-175. DOI: 10.1016/j.bodyim.2005.03.001

[76] Griffiths S, Mond JM, Murray SB, et al. Young peoples' stigmatizing attitudes and beliefs about anorexia nervosa and muscle dysmorphia. The International Journal of Eating Disorders. 2014;**47**(2):189-195

[77] Campbell K, Peebles R. Eating disorders in children and adolescents: State of the art review. Pediatrics. 2014;**134**(3):582-592

[78] Iwajomo T, Bondy SJ, de Oliveira C, et al. Excess mortality associated with eating disorders: Population-based cohort study. The British Journal of Psychiatry. 2020;**219**:1-7. DOI: 10.1192/bjp.2020.197

[79] Himmerich H, Hotopf M, Shetty H, et al. Psychiatric comorbidity as a risk factor for the mortality of people with bulimia nervosa. Social Psychiatry and Psychiatric Epidemiology. 2019;**54**:813-821

[80] Edakubo S, Fushimi K. Mortality and risk assessment for anorexia nervosa in acute-care hospitals: A nationwide administrative database analysis. BMC Psychiatry. 2020;**20**:19

[81] Pettersen G, Wallin K, Björk T. How do males recover from eating disorders? An interview study. BMJ Open. 2016;**6**(8):e010760. DOI: 10.1136/bmjopen-2015-010760

[82] American Psychiatric Association, editor. Treatment of patients with eating disorders. In: APA Practice Guidelines for the Treatment of Psychiatric Disorders: Comprehensive Guidelines and Guideline Watches. 3rd ed. Arlington, VA, USA: American Psychiatric Association; 2006

[83] Aigner M, Treasure J, Kaye W, Kasper S. The WFSBP task force on eating disorders world Federation of Societies of biological psychiatry (WFSBP) guidelines for the pharmacological treatment of eating disorders. The World Journal of Biological Psychiatry. 2011;**12**:400-443. DOI: 10.3109/15622975.2011.602720

[84] National Guideline Alliance (UK). Eating Disorders: Recognition and Treatment. Available from: https://www.nice.org.uk/guidance/ng69/ [Accessed: October 1, 2018]

[85] Kinnaird E, Norton C, Pimblett C, Stewart C, Tchanturia K. "There is nothing there for guys". Do men with eating disorders want treatment adaptations? A qualitative study. Eating and Weight Disorders. 2019;**24**(5):845-852. DOI: 10.1007/s40519-019-00770-0

[86] Dearden A, Mulgrew KE. Service provision for men with eating issues in Australia: An analysis of organizations', practitioners', and men's experiences. Australian Social Work. 2013;**66**(4):590-606. DOI: 10.1080/0312407X.2013.778306

[87] Arnow KD, Feldman T, Fichtel E, Lin IH, Egan A, Lock J, et al.

A qualitative analysis of male eating disorder symptoms. Eating Disorders. 2017;**25**(4):297-309. DOI: 10.1080/10640266.2017.1308729

[88] Bjork T, Wallin K, Pettersen G. Male experiences of life after recovery from an eating disorder. Eating Disorders. 2012;**20**(5):460-468. DOI: 10.1080/10640266.2012.7 15529

[89] Andersen A. Males and Eating Disorders. New York: Brunner/Mazel; 1990

[90] Bulik CM, Sullivan PF, Tozzi F, et al. Prevalence, heritability, and prospective risk factors for anorexia nervosa. Archives of General Psychiatry. 2006;**63**:305-312

Chapter 5

Dietary Patterns

Amra Ćatović

Abstract

Dietary patterns are defined as the quantities, proportions, variety, or combination of different foods, drinks, and nutrients in diets, and the frequency with which they are habitually consumed. Many social, demographic, and individual factors can have influence dietary patterns. A variety of food choices may benefit or harm health over time. Inappropriate dietary patterns are associated with risk of negative consequences in terms of diet-related chronic diseases, like cardiovascular disease, obesity, type 2 diabetes, and/or cancer. Dietary restriction behaviors can result in eating disorders including anorexia nervosa, bulimia nervosa, and binge eating disorder. Diet patterns are usually fairly well established, but they can change. Understanding of human nutrition can help to create eating patterns that help to achieve and maintain a healthy weight, reduce the risk of developing chronic diseases, and promote good health.

Keywords: dietary assessment, food choices, diet quality

1. Introduction

Health risk can be defined as "a factor that raises the probability of adverse health outcomes" [1]. Risk can be connected with the causal chain of events over time, consisting of socioeconomic factors, environmental and community conditions, and individual behavior. These risk roots may be used as intervention points [2]. Behaviors with a strong influence on health are tobacco use, alcohol consumption, physical activity and diet, sexual practices, and disease screening [3]. An essential factor of human physical and mental development is diet. It is fundamental to human health and wellbeing across the lifespan [4].

Diet refers to the foods and beverages a person consumes, eats and drinks. Specific kind of diet is designed with the types of foods and beverages a person chooses, like vegetarian diet, a weight-loss diet. Thus, the term diet does not mean a restrictive food plan associated with weight loss. Dietary patterns are defined as the amounts, proportions, variety, or combination of different foods, beverages, and nutrients in the diet, and the frequency with which they are commonly consumed. Many social, demographic, and individual factors can influence dietary patterns. Not individual food selections, but the balance of foods selected over time can benefit or harm health [5].

Deterioration of health is associated with inadequate nutrition. The term 'nutritional disorders' covers a wide range of conditions that are primarily nutritional or nutrition is an important factor in their etiology. They may include deficiencies or excesses in the diet, chronic diseases that have been stimulated by a dietary component, as well as developmental abnormalities in which diet has no role in etiology, but for which specific dietary intervention is an essential part of management (e.g., phenylketonuria), the interaction of foods and nutrients with drugs, food allergies. Eating disorders are not primarily nutritional disorders, but have important nutritional effects and significant metabolic consequences [6].

The medical and psychiatric consequences of eating disorders are numerous. Some consequences can be reversed with weight restoration and resumption of normal eating behaviors. On the other hand, other complications, such as low bone mineral density (BMD), can persist after disease resolution causing is associated prolonged increased fracture risk [7]. Some form of ED can progress in severe obesity [8].

Eating disorders can affect people of all body weights and shapes. They can occur even in people, who look healthy, such as athletes. The origin of eating disorders has not been fully elucidated. Risk factors for all eating disorders involve a combination of genetic, biological, behavioral, psychological, and social issues [9]. These factors may interact differently in different people, causing specific dietary behaviors.

Psychometric test, so called the Eating Attitudes Test (EAT-26) is in use to identify the risk of eating disorders based on attitudes, feelings and behaviors related to eating. It is the most widely used standardized test, focused to examine socio-cultural factors in the development and maintenance of eating disorders. There is children's version of the eating attitude test applicable in patients as young as 8 years old [10, 11]. With developing diagnostic criteria avoidant/restrictive food intake disorder can be distinguished from anorexia nervosa, bulimia nervosa, and binge-eating disorder [12].

Traditionally, inadequate nutrition has been simplified to identify health outcome primarily associated with a single nutrient or food. In last two decades, the focus for quantifying dietary exposures has shifted from single nutrients or foods to dietary patterns as dietary patterns can be more closely associated with overall health status and disease risk than consumption of individual foods or nutrients [13]. To have insight into overall diet it is necessary to analysis not only the foods, food groups, and nutrients, but also their combination and variety; and the frequency and quantity with which they are habitually consumed [14].

Analyzing food consumption as dietary patterns may provide a comprehensive approach to disease prevention or treatment. It can enhance conceptual understanding of human dietary practice, and provide guidance for nutrition intervention and education. The overall patterns of dietary intake might be easy for the public to interpret or translate into diets. Therefore, an emphasis on foods and beverages has improved translation to dietary recommendations for the general population [13, 14].

2. Dietary assessment methods

It is difficult to measure human behavior, especially to measure dietary exposures and capture the effects of eating behaviors. Diet intake of humans is assessed by objective observation and subjective report.

Objective observation can be done using a duplicate diet approach or food consumption record. Duplicate diet approach with direct analysis gives actual intake information throughout a specific period. Inherent strength is possibility of measurement of dietary exposures (e.g., environmental contaminants), but it not suitable for large-scale studies. Food consumption record is objective observation that ought to be done by trained staff at the household level. It obtains actual intake information throughout a specific period, but on individual level dietary consumption is not accurate. It is method of choice for those with low literacy or those who prepare most meals at home, and it is not suitable among those frequently eat outside the home [15].

Subjective assessment is possible using real-time recording (food diaries) or methods of recall. Self-reported recall methods can be in form of open-ended surveys such as 24 hours dietary recall - 24HR, dietary record - DR, dietary history since early life, or closed-ended surveys including food frequency questionnaire (FFQ). 24-Hour dietary recall uses open-ended questionnaires. It ought to be administered by a trained interviewer to obtain actual intake information over the previous 24 hours. However, there is possible recall bias as well as possible interviewer bias. Dietary record is subjective measure based on use of open-ended, self- administered questionnaires, so there is relatively large respondent burden (literacy and high motivation required, possible under-reporting). This method provides detailed intake data throughout a specific period. Dietary history has two parts: open- and closed-ended questionnaires administered by a trained interviewer. By this method, it is possible to assess usual dietary intake over a relatively long period [15].

Widely used direct assessment of dietary intake is FFQ. FFQ can has self- or interviewer- administered format. It is method of choice for large epidemiological studies to assess usual dietary intake estimated over a relatively long period (e.g., 6 months or 1 year). As diet can be influenced by social or individual factors, the FFQ should be developed specifically according to the interests of the research. FFQ can be food-based or dish-based, and focus may be on the intake of specific nutrients, or dietary exposures related to a certain disease. Semi-quantitative FFQs collecting data on the average portion sizes are in a closed format, and the simple FFQs that solely asks about the frequency or quantitative FFQs that queries about the amount of food consumption are based on completely open-ended questions [15, 16].

2.1 Meal patterns

To capture the interaction of nutrients and bioactive compounds within the whole diet, as people consume combinations of foods as meals and snacks, it is important to analyze meal patterns. To analyze contributions of meal patterns (also referred to as eating patterns) to energy and nutrient intakes and overall diet quality first the characterization, definition and measurement of 'meals' ought to be described. Meal may mean different things according cultural background, so different dimensions of meal patterns are in use to standardized criteria (for example, time-of day, number of hot/cold eating events). A main meal (for example, breakfast, lunch or dinner) or a smaller-sized meal (for example, supper or snack) are used to describe individuals' eating patterns. The terms 'eating occasion' (EO) or 'eating event' are used in defining any occasion where food or drink is consumed, so incorporates all meal types. A minimum energy criterion as part of the meal definition also can be included. According to this criterion, EO is only treated as an EO if it contributes a minimum amount of energy (for example, 210 kJ). The different definitions of an EO greatly affected the results of the association between eating frequency and BMI.

Meals are multidimensional and can be classified according to three constructs: (1) patterning (for example, frequency, spacing, regularity, skipping, timing); (2) format (for example, types of food combinations, sequencing of foods, nutrient profile/content); and (3) context (for example, eating with others or with the family, eating in front of the television or out of the home). However, due to the limited dietary assessment methods available, most research has focused on meal patterning [17].

Two major eating patterns were identified, which were qualitatively similar across the two FFQs and the diet records. So called 'prudent pattern' is characterized by a higher intake of vegetables, fruits, legumes, whole grains, and fish, whereas so called 'western pattern', is characterized by a higher intake of processed meat, red meat, butter, high-fat dairy products, eggs, and refined grains [14].

The methods of choice to assess meals are food diaries and 24 h recalls with collection data on time of eating, and contextual information (for example, location of eating, presence of others), as well as self-identified meals. FFQ provide estimates of the frequency and types of foods that are usually consumed, and there is need for additional questionnaires to collect information on meal patterns [15].

There are some modifications of assessing eating patterns included in The Eating Disorder Examination (EDE). Besides questions related to meal frequency (breakfast, lunch, and evening meal) and snack frequency (midmorning, afternoon and evening), there are those assesing binge eating or purging behaviors (frequency of self-induced vomiting, laxative misuse, diuretic misuse, driven exercise, fasting, subjective and objective meassure of binge eating episodes) [18].

Evaluation of the eating behaviors patients ought to include analysis of 1) nutrient intake (protein, fat, carbohydrates, vitamins, and minerals) 2) dietary quality (nutrient density, percentage of dietary energy derived from the macronutrients protein, fat, and carbohydrates), and 3) food groups as sources for the macronutrients.

Dietary variables are quantitative and qualitative. The quantitative variables include energy and nutrients intake (weight units), and nutrient density per 4.2 MJ/1000 kcal. The qualitative variables are the relative distribution of energy between macronutrients (E%), the selection of food items and food groups, as well as calculation of nutrients per their sources [19].

2.2 Diet quality index

Diet quality index is the most common measure used to assess overall diet quality. It is constructed on the basis of prevailing dietary recommendations, thus it is a summary score of the degree to which an individual's diet conforms to specific dietary recommendations. It reflects an individual's adherence to the dietary guidelines for the country of the sample population (for example, the Healthy Eating Index (HEI), and the Dietary Guidelines Index (DGI)), or adherence to other dietary recommendation: a traditional Mediterranean diet score; Dietary Approaches to Stop Hypertension diet score; a dietary approach to prevent heart disease diet score (Optimal Macronutrient Intake Trial to Prevent Heart Disease score) [14].

3. Eating patterns in ED

Main characteristic of anorectics eating behavior is a restriction of overall food intake, while vomiting/purging and intermittent starvation of bulimics is main mechanism of avoiding weight gain. The most commonly findings of food restriction are specific carbohydrate avoidance and, to a lesser degree, fat exclusion. However, anorectics and bulimics differ from each other with regard to food consumption patterns. Bulimics avoid bread and cereals, so they have less of their protein, fat, and carbohydrate energy from the bread/cereal group. On the other hand, anorectics prefer bread and cereals, at the same time trying to eliminate fat from their diets. Bread and cereals are thus the distinguishing feature between the ED groups.

The bread/cereal avoiding can be explain with bulimics attitude that carbohydrates from bread and cereals are particularly "fattening". Even their fear of carbohydrates, their diet contains a substantial proportion of carbohydrates from fruits and vegetables. Mostly, bulimics rate vegetables, fruit, lean meat as "safe", while cookies, bread, cakes, and fried are consider as "forbidden" foods. Consequence of this is that if the bulimic eats anything outside her preestablished dietary "allowance," she immediately resorts to binge eating. As the food choice among bulimics has often been demonstrated to be very narrow the non-purged diet consisted mainly of salads and diet sodas.

Anorectics on the other hand, have often been found to eat the same food every day, with explicated fear of "fatty" products [19, 20].

3.1 Eating patterns in individuals with anorexia nervosa

The mean generalization of AN is caloric restriction that resulted in weight loss. Restriction is greater during the more severe phases of the disorder. Beyond this restriction great variability in the diet patterns can be found. A regular meal and snack pattern can have approximately six eating episodes per day, in form of three meals and three snacks per day. Mostly, regular meals pattern is associated with a high-quality diet but restricted calorie. Inadequate calories during each eating episode are due to nature of insufficient quantities, or low caloric density food choices. This mainly rigid dietary pattern is caracteristic of restrictive type AN. Irregular eating patterns have fewer eating episodes on purge-only days, and more eating episodes on binge days (with or without purging) [16, 17]. Thus, less regular eating patterns are associated with loss of control eating. Meals are skipped with long intervals without eating at binge eating/purging type AN. Those with the BE/P type consume breakfast and dinner significantly less often than those with restricting type, and consume mid-morning snack and mid-afternoon sack significantly less often than those with restricting type. Among those with AN-BE/P, skipping dinner is associated with a greater number of binge eating episodes, while skipping breakfast is associated with a greater number of purging episodes. It may be the main mechanism associated with the development and maintenance of binge eating and purging. This mechanism suggests that dietary restraint leads to binge eating, which may lead to purging, and this in turn leads to a vicious cycle of increased efforts to restrict eating again. There is possibility that AN-BE/P often have higher eating disorder severity, more co-morbidities and worse prognosis than patients with AN-R [18].

Beside caloric restriction stereotyped food choices are characteristic of AN. Some food groups are chosen less often like bread and cereals, meat, cured meats, fatty foods, sweet foods and fried foods, but vegetables are chosen more often. Diet intake analyze has shown that restrictive anorexic females have a lower macronutrients intake than do healthy people, and illness duration specialy negatively correlats with the amount of fat in the diet. On the other hand, the relationship between unsaturated and saturated fats (MUFA + PUFA/SFA) is not significantly different between patients and healthy people. There are significant differences in some micronutrients content between the groups. There is tendency of lower intake of vitamin A and vitamin C, as well as sodium, phosphorus, zinc, copper, and selenium. It is established that, compared to controls, lower proportion of patients reached the DRI for thiamine, vitamin B6, calcium, iron and copper, although a higher proportion of patients reached the DRI for folate. Not only the majority of patients do not reach the DRI for pantothenic acid, folate, vitamin D, calcium, magnesium, iron, iodine and zinc, but that something similar occurs among healthy people [21, 22].

Not only AN, but avoidant/restrictive food intake disorder (ARFID) represents with avoidant or restrictive eating, but it is clearly different from AN. In patients with ARFID there are no disturbed cognitions about weight and/or shape, or a wish to lose weight. There are similar physical signs and symptoms as at AN patients, due to semi-starvation, like weight loss or lack of weight gain, nutritional deficiencies, reliance on tube feeding or oral nutritional supplements and/or disturbances in psychosocial functioning. On the other hand, ARFID patients are younger than AN patients and have a greater percentage of males. There are specific behaviors and symptoms in the ARFID group, including food avoidance, decreased appetite, abdominal pain, and emetophobia. While the degree of malnutrition is similar to that of patients with AN, those with ARFID have a greater dependence on nutritional supplements, fears of vomiting and/or choking, and texture/sensory issues pertaining to food. It can be explained by body preoccupation with somatic concerns. Some children express fears of physical illness due to issues related to shape/weight, e.g. high cholesterol and/or obesity leading to heart isease, either because of personal experiences with relatives or information in their school curriculum. Sometimes, worries about being fat, can be connected with events in the family's medical history, like recent myocardial infarction at an overweight relative. This event can be processed making illogical associations based on the cognitive developmental stage. This knowledge may then trigger restrictive eating behaviors. Thorough history-taking can often elicit this information [23].

3.2 Eating patterns in individuals with bulimia

The bulimics eating pattern can be described as intermittent starvation (i.e. non-purged diet during the restrictive or compensatory phase), interrupted by bouts of binge eating [18]. In the single-course normal meal, bulimics eat less on average than healthy nonbulimics. In patients with BN, objective food consumption ranges, in a sence of total energy consumption, as well as of energy intake per binge episode and the frequency of binge episodes. There is significant difference in the calories consumed by patients with BN during binge episodes compared to nonbinge meals [24, 25].

Thus, objective food consumption in a laboratory setting ranged from 7101 to 9360 kcal per 24 h and from 3030 to 4479 kcal per binge episode. However, subjective food records showed total energy consumption to range from 3117 to 4275 kcal per day and from 1173 to 2415 kcal per binge episode [22].

Even energy deprivation and malnutrition are often thought to be key factors in the maintenance of bulimia nervosa, it is unclear how much energy is actually available to BN patients' metabolism because the contribution of food consumed during binge eating is hard to evaluated [26].

3.3 Differences in binge behavior between bulimia nervosa and binge-eating disorder subjects

Binge eating is defined as the consumption of a large amount of food in a short period of time accompanied by a sense of lack of control over eating [12].

Binge eating has historically been associated with bulimia nervosa and the bulimia nervosa subjects eat more than BED subjects when presented with the same types of foods. It can be explained with fact that they allow themselves to purge following a binge. The frequency of binge episodes among individuals with BN ranged from 5.7 to 10.9 episodes per week, while the frequency of binge episodes among BED ranges from 10.7 to 17 episodes per 28 days [25].

Bulimics consumed increased caloric intake mainly because 37% of their meals were greater than 1000 calories. The binge foods consisted primarily of sweet desserts and snacks with a high fat content. This is connected with the avoidance of forbidden sugar and carbohydrate foods during nonbinge periods so cravings for these foods are reflected in their binges.

Thus, the binges of bulimics are higher in carbohydrates and sugar than those of individuals with BED. Generally, those with BED eat more fat, less protein, and an equal amount of carbohydrates when compared to nonbinge eaters what can be associated with their preference to choose foods eaten at a meal for binges [27, 28].

A disruption of circadian feeding patterns in sense that large meals are consumed mostly during the afternoon and evening have been seen at BN and BED. According to the diagnostic criteria, individuals with NES (night eating syndrome) should consume at least 25% of their total caloric intake after the evening meal. However, a delay in the circadian pattern of food intake (NES) may not be simply a variant of BED or BN but rather a separate entity that may lead to a more severe disorder [25].

4. Conclusions

Two EDs, anorexia nervosa (AN) and bulimia nervosa (BN), have historically been the primary EDs of focus. The DSM-5 updated diagnostic criteria for these disorders added two more: binge-eating disorder (BED) and avoidant/restrictive food intake disorder (ARFID) [12, 29].

Based on past versions of the DSM over 50% of patients met criteria for Eating Disorder Not Otherwise Specified (EDNOS). Recognition new disorders makes possibility to take a developmental, or life-span, approach to all disorders.

Patients with ARFID are less likely to report typical ED symptoms, e.g. purging behaviors and excessive exercise. They are younger, and a higher likelihood of being male. Children and adolescents with ARFID are more likely to present at a younger age with significant weight loss or failure to gain appropriate weight, are more dependent on oral or enteral nutritional supplementation, and have significantly more fears of choking and/or vomiting, and texture and/or sensitivity issues regarding food. They do not have body image distortion. However, some of them have body preoccupation with somatic concerns. Thus, evaluation of a young patient with possible ARFID versus AN, include probe about body concerns that need to be distinguished from body image distortion [23].

Disturbances in eating patterns is main characteristic of EDs. Dietary behaviors differ across the eating disorder diagnostic spectrum. For identification and classification of each EDs, it is important to define the associated eating patterns. Individuals with AN typically follow rigid dietary behaviors in meaning their meal times are fixed, they reduce portion sizes, they choose low caloric food. On the other hand, individuals with BN and BED tend to have more chaotic and inconsistent dietary behaviors and greater intra-individual variability. When they are not engaging in binge eating, individuals with AN-BE/P and BN have been found to attempt to restrict their caloric intake for the purpose of weight control, whereas individuals with BED have been found to be less likely to reduce their food consumption outside of binge eating with a slight tendency towards overeating [30].

The detailed description of the disturbances in eating behavior not only helps to identify diagnostic criteria associated with each disorder, but also provide a foundation for the development of treatment interventions [29]. Individuals who restrict caloric intake or consume meals and snacks with irregular frequency tend to engage in more frequent binge eating episodes. An irregular meal pattern of less than three meals a day is associated with more binge-eating episodes Specific dietary restriction behaviors, like reducing caloric intake by reducing portion sizes can increase risk for binge eating behaviors. Thus, it is important to identify dietary restriction behaviors that are associated with the onset of binge eating to cease it. A decrease in dietary restriction is a critical component for a successful reduction of binge eating behaviors across eating disorder diagnoses [30].

Conflict of interest

The author declares that she has no competing interests.

Abbreviations

24HR	24 hours dietary recall
AN	anorexia nervosa
AN/BN	anorectic bulimics
BE/P	binge eating/purging
BMI	body mass index
BN	bulimia nervosa
BMD	bone mineral density
DSM	Diagnostic and Statistical Manual of Mental Disorders
DGI	Dietary Guidelines Index
DR	dietary record
DRI	dietary reference intakes
EAT-26	Eating Attitudes Test
ED	eating disorder
EDE	Eating Disorder Examination
EDNOS	Eating Disorder Not Otherwise Specified
EO	eating occasion or eating event
FFQ	food frequency questionnaire
HEI	Healthy Eating Index
MUFAs	monounsaturated fatty acids
NES	night eating syndrome
PUFAs	polyunsaturated fatty acids
SFAs	saturated fatty acids

Author details

Amra Ćatović
Faculty of Medicine, Department of Hygiene, University of Sarajevo, Sarajevo, Bosnia and Herzegovina

*Address all correspondence to: amra.catovic@mf.unsa.ba

References

[1] World Health Organization. Global Health Risks: Mortality and Burden of Disease Attributable to Selected Major Risk Factors. World Health Organization, Geneva; 2009

[2] Commission on Social Determinants of Health. Closing the Gap in a Generation: Health Equity through Action on the Social Determinants of Health. World Health Organization, Geneva; 2008

[3] Institute of Medicine. Health and Behavior; the Interplay of Biological, Behavioral, and Societal Influences. Washington, DC: National Academy Press; 2001

[4] World Health Organization. Diet, Nutrition and the Prevention of Chronic Diseases. Technical Report Series No. 916. World Health Organization, Geneva; 2003

[5] Whitney EN, Rolfes SR. Understanding Nutrition. 15th ed. Boston: Cengage; 2017. pp. 3-69

[6] Ayling RM. Nutritional disorders and their management. In: Marshall WJ, Lapsley M, Day A, et al., editors. Clinical Biochemistry Metabolic and Clinical Aspects. Edinburgh: Elsevier; 2014. pp. 200-213

[7] Drabkin A, Rothman MS, Wassenaar E, Mascalo M, Mehler PS. Assessment and clinical management of bone disease in adults with eating disorders: A review. Journal of Eating Disorders. 2017;**5**:42

[8] Agüera Z, Lozano-Madrid M, Mallorquí-Bagué N, Jiménez-Murcia S, Menchón JM, Fernández-Aranda F. A review of binge eating disorder and obesity. Neuropsychiatrie. 2021;**35**:57-67

[9] National Institutes of Mental Health. Eating disorders. About More than Food. NIH Publication No. 21-MH-4901 Revised. National Institutes of Mental Health, Bethesda; 2021

[10] Garner DM, Olmsted MP, Bohr Y, Garfinkel PE. The eating attitudes test: Psychometric features and clinical correlates. Psychological Medicine. 1982;**12**(4):871-878

[11] Maloney MJ, McGuire JB, Daniels SR. Reliability testing of a children's version of the eating attitude test. Journal of the American Academy of Child and Adolescent Psychiatry. 1988;**27**(5):541-543

[12] American Psychiatric Association. Diagnostic and Statistical Manual of Mental Disorders. Fifth ed. Arlington, VA: American Psychiatric Association; 2013

[13] Committee DGA. Scientific Report of the 2020 Dietary Guidelines Advisory Committee: Advisory Report to the Secretary of Agriculture and the Secretary of Health and Human Services. Washington, DC: U.S. Department of Agriculture, Agricultural Research Service; 2020

[14] Hu FB. Dietary pattern analysis: A new direction in nutritional epidemiology. Current Opinion in Lipidology. 2002;**13**:3-9

[15] Shim JS, Oh K, Kim HC, et al. Dietary assessment methods in epidemiologic studies. Epidemiology Health. 2014;**36**:e2014009

[16] Naska A, Lagiou A, Lagiou P. Dietary assessment methods in epidemiological research: Current state of the art

and future prospects [version 1; referees: 3 approved]. F1000Research. 2017;**6**(F1000 Faculty Rev):926

[17] Leech RM, Worsley A, Timperio A, McNaughton SA. Understanding meal patterns: Definitions, methodology and impact on nutrient intake and diet quality. Nutrition Research Reviews. 2015;**28**:1-21

[18] Elran-Barak R, Accurso EC, Goldschmidt AB, Sztainer M, Byrne C, Le Grange D. Eating patterns in youth with restricting and binge eating/purging type anorexia nervosa. The International Journal of Eating Disorders. 2014;**47**(8): 878-883

[19] Van der Ster WG, Norring C, Lennernas MA, Holmgren S. Food selection in anorectics and bulimics: Food items, nutrient content and nutrient density. Journal of the American College of Nutrition. 1995;**14**(3):271-277

[20] Van der Ster WG, Norring C, Holmgren S. Selective dieting patterns among anorectics and bulimics at the onset of eating disorders. European Eating Disorders Review. 1994;**2**(4):221-232

[21] Huse DM, Lucas AR. Dietary patterns in anorexia nervosa. The American Journal of Clinical Nutrition. 1984;**40**:251-254

[22] Jáuregui-Lobera I, Bolaños-Ríos P. Choice of diet in patients with anorexia nervosa. Nutrición Hospitalaria. 2009;**24**(6):682-687

[23] Nicely TA, Lane-Loney S, Masciulli E, Hollenbeak CS, Ornstein RM. Prevalence and characteristics of avoidant/ restrictive food intake disorder in a cohort of young patients in day treatment for eating disorders. Journal of Eating Disorders. 2014;**2**(1):21-28

[24] Walsh BT, Kissileff HR, Casidy SM, Dantzic S. Eating behavior of women with bulimia. Archives of General Psychiatry. 1989;**46**:54-58

[25] Latzer Y, Yutal AE, Givon M, Kabakov O, Alon S, Zuckerman-Levin N, et al. Dietary patterns of patients with binge eating disorders with and without night eating. Eating and Weight Disorders. 2020;**25**(2):321-328

[26] Alpers GW, Tuschen-Caffier B. Energy and macronutrient intake in bulimia nervosa. Eating Behavior. 2004;**5**(3):241-249

[27] Weltzin TE, Hsu LG, Pollice C, Kaye WH. Feeding patterns in bulimia nervosa. Biological Psychiatry. 1991;**30**:1093-1110

[28] Fitzgibbon ML, Blackman LR. Binge eating disorder and bulimia nervosa: Differences in the quality and quantity of binge eating episodes. The International Journal of Eating Disorders. 2000;**27**(2):238-243

[29] Heaner MK, Timothy WB. A history of the identification of the characteristic eating disturbances of bulimia nervosa, binge eating disorder and anorexia nervosa. Appetite. 2013;**71**:445-448

[30] Elran-Barak R, Sztainer M, Goldschmidt AB, Crow SJ, Peterson CB, Hill LL, et al. Dietary restriction behaviors and binge eating in anorexia nervosa, bulimia nervosa and binge eating disorder: Trans-diagnostic examination of the restraint model. Eating Behaviors. 2015;**18**:192-196

Section 3

Social Networks and Eating Disorders

Chapter 6

Perspective Chapter: Social Networks and Eating Disorders - Beauty and the Beast?

José María Otín-del Castillo, José Vicente Martínez-Quiñones and Ignacio Jáuregui-Lobera

Abstract

Currently, social networks are part of the lives of adolescents, who make intensive use of them to relate to each other and to the world, making them a major factor in socialization. This has led to a great deal of scientific research on the influence of this means of communication in many areas of the life and development of adolescents, especially in the field of both physical and mental health. This paper reviews some relevant psychological phenomena associated with the use of social networks to understand their influence on adolescent behaviour; the main psychosocial risk factors for problematic internet use at this stage and their possible relationship with eating disorders based on recent research findings; as well as some proposals adopted within the European Union and in Spanish legislation for the control of harmful content on the Internet, especially those related to the advocacy of anorexia and bulimia, which until very recently escaped any possibility of control despite their importance for public health. Finally, we briefly discuss the potential of technology to implement these controls and present a research project for the detection and neutralization of apology of ED on Twitter, funded and implemented by the APE Foundation with the collaboration of the University of Zaragoza.

Keywords: social networks, eating disorders, problematic internet use, anorexia and bulimia advocacy

1. Introduction

The use of social media has experienced a growth boom in recent years, a trend that continues unstoppably. In April 2022, it is estimated that there will be 4.65 billion social network users, which represents 58.7% of the world's population [1]. The latest study on the impact of technology on adolescence conducted by UNICEF Spain in 2021, indicates that 98.5% of adolescents are registered on at least one social network [2]. The same study concludes that the use of screens is a non-negotiable contribution to adolescents, both socially and emotionally.

These data are important in view of the prevalence of eating disorders, whose target population in Spain is women aged 12–36 years, with a prevalence ranging from

4.1 to 6.4 % between 12 and 21 years; it is one of the three most frequent chronic diseases among adolescents, a population in which it appears at an increasingly younger age [3]. A recent review of the scientific literature found that adolescents are a risk group for the development of eating disorders and the media is a contributing factor to dysfunctional eating behaviour [4].

On the other hand, some psychological phenomena characteristic of the use of the internet and social networks such as the so-called echo chambers and filter bubbles have been the subject of research into their effects and the possible relationship between the use of social networks and eating disorders in adolescence; This, in turn, has led to a growing concern of government authorities to control harmful content related to anorexia and bulimia distributed on the internet [5] and has stimulated the development of legislative measures and technical-scientific lines of research aimed at this objective.

2. Echo chambers and filter bubbles

The term echo chamber refers to the cognitive isolation in a media space of the user of digital content, which has the power to enhance the messages emitted in that space [such as a website, a blog, or the wall of an Instagram profile] while shielding them from hypothetical refutation [6]. This phenomenon is based on the so-called confirmation and disconfirmation biases, whereby people unconsciously tend to preferentially seek out information consistent with their prior beliefs and expectations while ignoring data that contradicts them [7].

The filter bubble is essentially an echo chamber resulting from the application of content personalisation algorithms implemented by the platforms on which they are offered, based on the user's previous activity, with the aim of providing them with content that is more attractive, interesting and in line with their interests [8].

The main difference between the two phenomena lies in the type of choice made by the user, more active in the case of echo chambers and totally passive in the filter bubble, since the content becomes accessible to the user after a prior automatic process of data analysis that is beyond their control, and which replaces the active choices themselves.

Recent research has focused on the possible link between these phenomena and eating disorders. The filter bubble is strongly associated with social networks, allowing users to choose which accounts to follow and encouraging selective or limited exposure to certain content, feeding back certain beliefs and behaviours [9]. An example of this is content related to the idealised representation of excessively thin bodies ['thinspiration']; exposure to this content has been found to be related to the severity of symptoms in people with ED [10].

In a recent study [11] on sources of health misinformation on the Internet, including misinformation about eating disorders, the authors warned of the echo chamber effect that online anorexia and bulimia nervosa communities promoting pro-eating disorder identities have on their members. Another study [12] describes these communities as authentic shared worlds for their members, which support and sustain the epistemic and affective dimensions of anorexia nervosa, as well as the role they play in maintaining the disorder through their intersubjective dimension and echo chamber effect. Evidence has also been found for this effect on pro-anorexia communities on Twitter as opposed to communities that support efforts to recover from the disease. Members of pro-anorexia communities tend to interact more closely with each other than healthy communities, and their interactions are more characterised by negative emotions [13]. Online communities' characteristics of social networks such as Twitter and Facebook provide people at risk for an eating disorder with anonymity, social support and information related to the disease [14, 15].

3. Problematic use of the Internet and eating disorders

In Spain, according to the results of the aforementioned study [2], 33% of adolescents [mostly girls] are reported to be developing problematic use of the internet and social networks. Problematic internet use is used instead of the term addiction, as internet addiction is not currently scientifically defined as such in the main disease classification manuals, such as the DSM5 or the ICD-11. Moreover, the term problematic internet use is a neutral term that places the focus of the problem on the user and possible misuse of the internet rather than on the internet itself [16].

The International Association of Child and Adolescent Psychiatry and Allied Professionals [IACAPAP] defines this behaviour as an exaggerated preoccupation with Internet use, experienced as irresistible for longer periods of time than expected, and which is accompanied by significant distress or behavioural impairment caused by this abuse in the absence of other psychiatric pathology that could explain the excessive Internet use [17].

On the other hand, some of the psychological factors of vulnerability to problematic internet use [18, 19] are consistent with factors related to the risk of developing EDs [20–23], such as low self-esteem, body image dissatisfaction and mood disorders such as depression and anxiety.

Thus, it is easy to conclude that universal access to the internet by adolescents, problematic internet use and the coincidence of risk factors form the 'perfect storm' to consolidate the association between social network use and EDs, which has been the subject of research for more than a decade.

Some recent studies support different aspects of this association, such as the existence of a clear relationship between body image, body preoccupation, body dissatisfaction and EDs among adolescent female students [24]; the increased likelihood of presenting with CD due to the greater number and frequency of social media use [25]; the relationship between healthy eating communities on Instagram, their intensive use and the prevalence and increased symptoms of orthorexia in their members [9]; the existence of a significant direct relationship between the frequency of social media use and the risk of developing EDs [26]; the immediate negative effects on young women of exposure to pro-anorexia websites [27] or the relationship between problematic internet use and EDs [28–30].

4. The control of harmful online content: the case of the European Union and Spain

In addition to the problematic use of social networks by adolescents at risk of suffering or already affected by EDs, the control of harmful content related to these disorders has been a recurrent concern and a long-standing demand of all sectors involved in the fight against EDs, which have traditionally experienced with anguish how the apology of anorexia and bulimia are easily and abundantly available on the Internet since they cannot be criminally prosecuted as they are not considered criminal content.

In this respect, a clear distinction should be made between these and so-called harmful content. Illegal or criminal content is delimited in a civil or criminal law norm [mainly criminalised in criminal codes, or considered contrary to fundamental rights such as honour and self-image in civil law].

Harmful content, on the other hand, is content that is considered likely to cause physical or psychological harm to those who consume it, but is not defined as a crime in the Criminal Code or does not meet the requirements for punishability; and which is usually grouped together in so-called dangerous online communities [groups of people with common interests, their own identity on the Internet and difficult to control].

However, the consideration of harmful content does not have a clear reference, as may be the case with the conduct defined as a crime in the various criminal codes, and is imprecise and open to interpretation, which poses risks to legal certainty [31]. As early as 1996, the European Union alluded to the difficulty of identifying and classifying online content likely to harm minors and indicated that the consideration of harmful content depends on cultural differences and that each country must therefore decide where the, sometimes fine, line separating it from illegal content lies [32]. This issue has been a burden on the various attempts to solve the problem up to the present day. Meta, one of the giants of the social networks and owner of Facebook and Instagram, considers this issue one of the four 'key questions' that it develops in its recent white paper on the regulation of online content [33], alluding to the thorny relationship with fundamental rights such as freedom of expression and opinion, deriving the responsibility for content moderation to governments, given the complexity of its consideration as harmful [34].

However, UNICEF includes in the category of harmful content that may contribute to aggravate eating disorders such as anorexia and bulimia because of their capacity to harm the development or endanger the right to health of children and adolescents [35]. According to this conception, content such as advocacy of anorexia and bulimia, promoters of the lifestyle known as 'thinspiration' or similar groups and online communities of 'Pro Ana and Mia' movements and extreme diets, would therefore fall into this category.

References to the fight against harmful content have been constant in the European Union's internet regulatory framework since the first Communication mentioned above. In 2012, it mentioned the need to protect minors from illegal and harmful content in the 'European strategy on making the internet more suitable for children' [36]. In 2017, it called on online platforms to strengthen measures to combat illegal and harmful content online [37]. In 2018, it drew up a recommendation on measures to effectively combat illegal content online [38], and in 2020 it included this issue in its Proposal for a Regulation on the Digital Single Market for Digital Services, better known as the Digital Services Act [39].

In Spain, the most important initiative is Law 34/2002, of 11 July, on information society services and electronic commerce, which imposes on service providers the obligation to inform about existing tools for filtering and restricting access to certain Internet content and services that are unwanted or may be harmful to young people and children [40], subsequently supported by other legal regulations [41, 42]. However, the aforementioned legal vagueness of 'harmful content' prevented a real application of the law. An example of this is the Study on Social Networks approved by the Congress of Deputies in 2015 [43], which devotes a section in its operative part to harmful content and recommendations for its control, without defining it as such or even proposing its conceptualisation.

Various groups involved in the fight against EDs have been fighting for the clear legal regulation of harmful content on the internet related to these disorders. Thus, the APE Foundation in Spain, after several years of efforts in this regard, 2017 succeeded in presenting to the Aragonese Parliamentary Bureau a Proposition of Law, supported by all parliamentary groups, on the eradication of internet content and social networks harmful to EDs. The Dialogue Table for the Prevention of ED, co-led by the Catalan Consumer Agency and the Association Against Anorexia and Bulimia, achieved the modification of the Catalan Consumer Code in 2019 to include as a serious offence the activities of promotion, advertising, offer or any other activity that encourages or induces consumers to adopt habits related to eating disorders, such as anorexia and bulimia among others [44, 45].

This being the case, we had to wait until the publication of the new Organic Law 8/2021, of 4 June, on the comprehensive protection of children and adolescents against violence [46], to finally find a clear tool for the fight against harmful content related to EDs. This legal norm obliges public administrations to promote the implementation and use of parental control mechanisms to protect minors from the risk of exposure to this content [Art. 46], including the inclusion in the Penal Code of a new article 361 bis that punish 'the distribution or public dissemination through the Internet, telephone or any other information or communication technology of content specifically intended to promote or facilitate, among minors or persons with disabilities in need of special protection, the consumption of products, preparations or substances or the use of techniques for the ingestion or elimination of food products whose use is likely to generate a risk to people's health'.

This new criminal classification of the apology of ED is undoubtedly an important step forward in this area, although its practical application presents important difficulties, such as the fact that most of the people who produce, distribute or share this content belong precisely to the sector of the population it is intended to protect: young people and adolescents who suffer from one of these ED; or the progressive displacement of the publication of this content from websites to social networks and from these to instant messaging applications, where the control of the dissemination of content is very complicated.

5. The fight against ATTs on the Internet: some proposals

Given the difficulties of effective repressive control of harmful content related to ATTs by governmental authorities, measures to prevent and educate users about these risks seem more easily applicable, although their real effectiveness is unknown.

In 1999, the European Union established the so-called Safer Internet Plan, which under different names and in different phases evolved into the current initiative called 'Better Internet for Kids' [47], which includes help and information lines for children and adolescents on dangerous communities 'Pro-Ana' and 'Pro-Mía', and which in Spain is managed by the National Cybersecurity Institute [INCIBE] through its IS4K Internet Segura for Kids programme [48].

The most important Internet service providers have been implementing measures to control the dissemination of ATTs beyond the possibilities of active protection that users themselves can implement on their devices through the wide range of parental control applications and configurations available, with the introduction of specific algorithms for the establishment of filters for this content based on the creation of keyword dictionaries. Thus, when search engines detect these words or hashtags, they provide the user with a warning message about the risk of search-related posts and the link to help services in this respect, but still offer the possibility to access the searched content.

Similarly, they have implemented specific information about these disorders on their support pages, including help resources [49–51] and even directly prohibited the publication of content that promotes eating habits that may have adverse health consequences [52, 53].

In this line of the fight against harmful content on the Internet related to eating disorders, the APE Foundation for the prevention and eradication of EDs has promoted the development of a computer tool for the early detection of apology of EDs on Twitter in collaboration with the University of Zaragoza. The project, currently under development, is based on monitoring key hashtags using natural language processing techniques to identify harmful messages in the context of ATTs, allowing the detection of accounts that disseminate such content for reporting. It also includes a tool for analysing the interaction between active accounts, and identifying communities of users, which would help in the prevention and early detection of these disorders [54].

6. Conclusions

The internet and social networks have become powerful means of communication for adolescents. Problematic use of internet is related to a higher risk of suffering from these disorders in this population segment, which is why the control of harmful content related to the promotion of EDs is an objective of public administrations. However, the lack of legal definition of this content has hindered its possible control. Nevertheless, the European Union is working on the issue through different legislative instruments and Spain has recently criminalised these conducts, which, despite being a clear advance in the matter, poses significant difficulties in its practical application; therefore, in parallel, different areas have been working on measures for prevention, information and support for people affected by these disorders.

Acknowledgements

We thank APE Foundation for its interest in fighting against the spreading of eating disorders in the Media. Its activities aim to reduce the influence of those Media among adolescents, thus reducing the number of new eating disorders patients.

Conflict of interest

The authors declare no conflict of interest.

Author details

José María Otín-del Castillo, José Vicente Martínez-Quiñones
and Ignacio Jáuregui-Lobera*
APE Foundation, Zaragoza, Spain

*Address all correspondence to: ignacio-ja@teefonica.net

References

[1] Kepios. Global social media statistics — DataReportal – Global digital insights [cited 2022 Jul 26]. Available from: https://datareportal.com/social-media-users

[2] Andrade B, Guadix I, Rial A, Suárez F. Impacto de la tecnología en la adolescencia. Relaciones, riesgos y oportunidades. Madrid: UNICEF España; 2021

[3] Aragón (Spain) Eating Disorders Association. Statistics on eating disorders 2020 [cited 2022 Jul 26]. Available from: https://www.tca-aragon.org/2020/06/01/estadisticas-sobre-los-tca/

[4] Bittar C, Soares A. Mídia e comportamento alimentar na adolescência. Cadernos Brasileiros de Terapia Ocupacional. 2020;**28**(1):291-308

[5] Rodríguez O, Rodríguez MC. Control de contenidos en el Internet: Una realidad que puede ser vista como una amenaza. Revista de Derecho, Comunicaciones y Nuevas Tecnologías. 2005;**1**:17-51

[6] Nguyen CT. Echo chambers and epistemic bubbles. Episteme. 2020;**17**(2):141-161

[7] Plous S. The Psychology of Judgment and Decision Making. New York: McGraw-Hill; 1993

[8] Arguedas MR, Robertson CT, Fletcher R, Nielsen RK. Echo Chambers, Filter Bubbles, and Polarisation: a Literature Review. Oxford: University of Oxford; 2022

[9] Turner PG, Lefevre CE. Instagram use is linked to increased symptoms of orthorexia nervosa. Eating and Weight Disorders - Studies on Anorexia, Bulimia and Obesity. 2017;**22**(2):277-284

[10] Griffiths S, Castle D, Cunningham M, Murray SB, Bastian B, Barlow FK. How does exposure to thinspiration and fitspiration relate to symptom severity among individuals with eating disorders? Evaluation of a proposed model. Body Image. 2018;**27**:187-195

[11] Suarez-Lledó V, Álvarez-Gálvez J. Prevalence of health misinformation on social media: Systematic review [Preprint]. Journal of Medical Internet. 2021 Jan 20;**23**(1):e17187. DOI: 10.2196/17187

[12] Osler L, Krueger J. ProAna Worlds: Affectivity and Echo Chambers Online. Topoi 2021. DOI: 10.1007/s11245-021-09785-8. [Accepted 19 November 2021, Published 12 December 2021]

[13] Wang T, Brede M, Ianni A, Mentzakis E. Social interactions in online eating disorder communities: A network perspective. PLOS One. 2018;**13**(7):e0200800

[14] Arseniev-Koehler A, Lee H, McCormick T, Moreno MA. Proana: Pro-eating disorder socialization on twitter. Journal of Adolescent Health. 2016;**58**(6):659-664

[15] Saunders JF, Eaton AA. Snaps, selfies, and shares: How three popular social media platforms contribute to the sociocultural model of disordered eating among young women. Cyberpsychology, Behavior, and Social Networking. 2018;**21**(6):343-354

[16] Matute H. Adicción, abuso o uso problemático de internet. In: Echeburúa, E (Coord). Abuso de Internet ¿antesala para la adicción al juego de azar online? (pp. 19-35). Madrid: Editorial Pirámide. 2016

[17] Chang JPC, Hung CC. Problematic use of Internet. In: International Association for Child and Adolescent Psychiatry and Allied Professions (IACAPAP). e-Textbook of Child and Adolescent Mental Health. 2019. Chapter H-6

[18] Becoña Iglesias E. Factores de riesgo y de protección en el uso problemático de internet. In: Echeburúa, E (Coord.) Abuso de Internet ¿antesala para la adicción al juego de azar online? (pp. 36-63). Madrid: Editorial Pirámide. 2016

[19] Hay P, Morris J. Eating disorders. In: International Association for Child and Adolescent Psychiatry and Allied Professions (IACAPAP). e-Textbook of Child and Adolescent Mental Health. 2019. Chapter H-1

[20] Borrego Hernando O. Tratamiento de los trastornos de la conducta alimentaria: Anorexia y Bulimia. Información Terapéutica del Sistema Nacional de Salud. 2000;**24**:44-50

[21] Brown Z, Tiggemann M. Attractive celebrity and peer images on Instagram: Effect on women's mood and body image. Body Image. 2016;**19**:37-43

[22] Keel PK, Forney KJ. Psychosocial risk factors for eating disorders. International Journal of Eating Disorders. 2013;**46**(5):433-439

[23] Trottier K, Polivy Jy, Herman CP. Effects of exposure to thin and overweight peers: Evidence of social comparison in restrained and unrestrained eaters. Journal of Social and Clinical Psychology. 2007;**26**(2):155-172

[24] Aparicio-Martínez P, Perea-Moreno AJ, Martínez-Jiménez MP, Redel-Macías MD, Pagliari C, Vaquero-Abellán M. Social media, thin-ideal, body dissatisfaction and disordered eating attitudes: An exploratory analysis. International Journal of Environmental Research and Public Health. 2019;**16**(21):4177

[25] Bernardo Arnal L. Relación entre el uso de redes sociales y trastornos de la conducta alimentaria. [Trabajo Fin de Grado no publicado]. Facultad de Medicina, Universidad Católica de Valencia San Vicente Mártir. Valencia: Universidad Católica San Vicente Martir. 2021. Available from: https://riucv.ucv.es/bitstream/handle/20.500.12466/1769/RELACI%C3%93N%20ENTRE%20EL%20USO%20DE%20REDES%20SOCIALES%20Y%20TRASTORNOS%20DE%20LA%20CONDUCTA%20ALIMENTARIA.pdf?sequence=1&isAllowed=y

[26] Ojeda-Martín A, López-Morales MP, Jáuregui-Lobera I, Herrero-Martín G. Uso de redes sociales y riesgo de padecer TCA en jóvenes. Journal of Negative and No Positive Results. 2021;**6**(10):1289

[27] Bardone-Cone AM, Cass KM. What does viewing a pro-anorexia website do? An experimental examination of website exposure and moderating effects. International Journal of Eating Disorders. 2007;**40**(6):537-548

[28] García Puertas D. Influencia del uso de Instagram sobre la conducta alimentaria y trastornos emocionales. Revisión sistemática. Revista española de comunicación en salud. 2020;**11**(2):244

[29] Ioannidis K, Taylor C, Holt L, Brown K, Lochner C, Fineberg NA, et al. Problematic usage of the internet and eating disorder and related psychopathology: A multifaceted, systematic review and meta-analysis. Neuroscience & Biobehavioral Reviews. 2021;**125**:569-581

[30] Kożybska M, Radlińska I, Czerw A, Dykowska G, Karakiewicz B. There are predictors of eating disorders among

internet use characteristics—A cross-sectional study on the relationship between problematic internet use and eating disorders. International Journal of Environmental Research and Public Health. 2021;**18**(19):10269

[31] Sánchez Bravo A. La regulación de los contenidos ilícitos y nocivos en Internet: Una propuesta desde la Unión Europea. Informática y Derecho: Revista Iberoamericana de derecho informático. Universidad Nacional de Educación a Distancia (UNED), Spain. 1998. pp. 27-29

[32] Comunicación de la Comisión al Consejo, al Parlamento Europeo, al Comité Económico y Social y al Comité de las Regiones. Contenidos ilícitos y nocivos en Internet, COM(96)487 final, 1996

[33] Bickert M. Charting a way forward on online content regulation. 2020. Available from: https://about.fb.com/news/2020/02/online-content-regulation/ [cited 2022 Jul 26]

[34] Bickert M. Trazando un Camino a seguir en la regulación de los contenidos online. 2020. Available from: https://about.fb.com/es/news/2020/02/trazando-un-camino-a-seguir-en-la-regulacion-de-los-contenidos-online/ [cited 2022 Jul 26]

[35] UNICEF. Educando en el derecho a la información: Contenidos falsos, nocivos e ilícitos. Available from: https://www.unicef.es/educa/blog/educando-derecho-informacion-contenidos-falsos-nocivos-ilicitos [cited 2022 Jul 26]

[36] European Strategy for a Better Internet for Children. Communication from the commission to the European Parliament, the council, the European economic and social committee and the committee of the regions. Document 52012DC0196. Available from: https://eur-lex.europa.eu/legal-content/es/TXT/?uri=CELEX:52012DC0196 [cited 2022 Jul 26]

[37] European Parliament. European Parliament resolution of 15 June 2017 on online platforms and the digital single market (2016/2276(INI)). Available from: https://www.europarl.europa.eu/doceo/document/TA-8-2017-0272_EN.html [cited 2022 Jul 26]

[38] Official Journal of the European Union | L 63/50. Commission Recommendation (EU) 2018/334 of 1 March 2018 on measures to effectively tackle illegal content online. Available from: https://eur-lex.europa.eu/legal-content/EN-ES/TXT/?from=ES&uri=CELEX%3A32018H0334 [cited 2022 Jul 26]

[39] Propuesta de reglamento del Parlamento Europeo y del Consejo relativo a un mercado único de servicios digitales (Ley de servicios digitales) y por el que se modifica la Directiva 2000/31/CE 15 December 2020. Available from: https://eur-lex.europa.eu/legal-content/ES/ALL/?uri=CELEX:52020PC0825#

[40] Ley 34/2002, de 11 de julio, de servicios de la sociedad de la información y de comercio electrónico. Boletín Oficial del Estado, 66, 12 July 2002

[41] Ley 9/2014, de 9 de mayo, General de Telecomunicaciones. Boletín Oficial del Estado, 114, 10 May 2014

[42] Real Decreto 2296/2004, de 10 de diciembre, por el que se aprueba el Reglamento sobre mercados de comunicaciones electrónicas, acceso a las redes y numeración. Boletín Oficial del Estado, 314, 30 December 2004

[43] Acuerdo de la Comisión de Interior relativo al Informe de la Subcomisión de Estudio sobre las Redes Sociales, 24 de marzo de 2015. Boletín Oficial del Estado, 643, 9 April 2015

[44] Ley 22/2010, de 20 de julio, del Código de consumo de Cataluña. Boletín Oficial del Estado, 196, 13 August 2010

[45] Apología de los TCA. Associació Contra l'Anorèxia i la Bulímia. 2020. Available from: https://www.acab.org/es/los-trastornos-de-conducta-alimentaria/que-son-los-tca/apologia-de-los-tca/

[46] Ley Orgánica 8/2021, de 4 de junio, de protección integral a la infancia y la adolescencia frente a la violencia. Boletín Oficial del Estado,134, 5 June 2021. Available from: https://www.boe.es/eli/es/lo/2021/06/04/8

[47] European Commission. A European strategy for a better internet for kids (BIK+), 2022. Available from: https://digital-strategy.ec.europa.eu/en/policies/strategy-better-internet-kids [cited 2022 Jul 26]

[48] Securekids. Secure Internet for Kids. Available from: https://www.is4k.es/de-utilidad/herramientas/securekids. [cited 2022 Jul 26]

[49] Instagram Help Center. About Eating Disorders. Available from: https://help.instagram.com/252214974954612/?helpref=hc_fnav [cited 2022 Jul 26]

[50] Facebook Help Service. What should I do if a friend has posted on Facebook that seems to indicate that they have an eating disorder?. Available from: https://es-es.facebook.com/help/230070543674737/?helpref=uf_share [cited 2022 Jul 26]

[51] Trastorno alimentario. 2021. TikTok. Available from: https://www.tiktok.com/safety/es-es/eating-disorder/

[52] Available from: https://www.tiktok.com/community-guidelines?lang=es#33

[53] Política contra suicidio o daño autoinfligido de Twitter | Ayuda de Twitter. 2021. Help Center. Available from: https://help.twitter.com/es/rules-and-policies/glorifying-self-harm

[54] Rey DR. Infraestructura software para el análisis de las interacciones en Twitter: Aplicación a la detección de trastornos de conducta alimentaria. [Trabajo Fin de Grado no publicado]. Departamento de Informática e Ingeniería de Sistemas, EINA. Zaragoza: Universidad de Zaragoza; 2020. Available from: https://webdiis.unizar.es/~ricardo/files/TFGs/AnalisisInteracciones TwitterDeteccionTCA.pdf